In Clinical Practice

For further volumes
http://www.springer.com/series/13483

David T. Huang • Travis Prinzi
Editors

Clinical Cardiac Electrophysiology in Clinical Practice

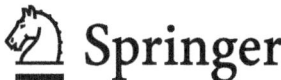 Springer

Editors
David T. Huang, MD
Department of Cardiology
University of Rochester
Medical Center
Rochester, NY
USA

Travis Prinzi, MD
Department of Cardiology
University of Rochester
Medical Center
Rochester, NY
USA

ISBN 978-1-4471-5432-7   ISBN 978-1-4471-5433-4   (eBook)
DOI 10.1007/978-1-4471-5433-4
Springer London Heidelberg New York Dordrecht

Library of Congress Control Number: 2014956969

*"To my wife Carlene
and our children Allison,
Claudia, and Samantha.
Thank you for all your
tolerance, commitment, and
love." – DH*

selected for use the latest and most relevant equipment and techniques for optimizing interventional electrophysiology.

Dr. Huang realized that there is remarkably little that has been written about the integrative technical details involved in day-to-day electrophysiology procedures, i.e., setting up and delivering approaches for arrhythmia mapping, describing diagnostic catheter maneuvering, highlighting effective ablative techniques, and substantiating the antiarrhythmic efficacy of what has been done and accomplished before the patient leaves the laboratory. This authoritative book emphasizes the practical aspects of establishing, delivering, and maintaining up-to-date laboratory approaches utilizing various technologies that have improved the treatment of patients with a spectrum of cardiac arrhythmias.

Clinical Cardiac Electrophysiology in Clinical Practice focuses on introductory electrophysiology with a comprehensive coverage of practical information that will be useful for new and established electrophysiologists, trainees and fellows, and support staff including nurses and physician assistants involved in electrophysiological procedures. The information in this book not only emphasizes the proven electrophysiological approaches that are currently useful and effective in arrhythmia management but it also provides insight into how to stay abreast of ongoing new and more effective techniques in the field.

In his *Aphorisms*, Sir William Osler stated that "When you have made and recorded the unusual or original observation, or when you have accomplished a piece of research in laboratory or ward, do not be satisfied with a verbal communication at a medical society. Publish it." We are fortunate that for those involved in clinical electrophysiology, this is exactly what Dr. David Huang and his associates have done.

Arthur J. Moss, MD
Bradford C. Berk, MD, PhD,
University of Rochester School of Medicine
and Dentistry, Rochester, NY, USA

Foreword

During the past 40 years, there has been a meaningful advancement in our diagnostic understanding of the mechanisms of various bradyarrhythmias, supraventricular and ventricular tachyarrhythmias, and pre-excitation syndromes. This new knowledge has developed during a proliferation of more effective techniques for the management of these arrhythmias, with increasing emphasis on radiofrequency ablation techniques at a time when the ineffectiveness and side effects of antiarrhythmic drugs have become more evident. The field of clinical electrophysiology has matured considerably within the twenty-first century with more sophisticated intracardiac mapping techniques that have permitted precise and focused ablative termination of previously considered refractory arrhythmias. These improved therapeutic approaches are now coupled with innovative technologies that reconstruct the dynamics of the arrhythmias within three-dimensional models of the heart—thus providing a unique visualization of the pattern of the disordered electrophysiological conduction pattern in the heart.

I have known Dr. David Huang well as a colleague and research investigator during the 16 years he has been at the University of Rochester Medical Center. At a personal level, he is dedicated to excellence in patient care—at the bedside, in the clinic, and in the electrophysiology laboratory. In brief, he is the clinician's clinician. Together with his skills as a clinician, he has created in Rochester an outstanding team of electrophysiologists who have provided effective approaches to the diagnosis and management of the full spectrum of cardiac arrhythmias. During this time, he has evaluated and

Contents

Contributors

Mehmet K. Aktas, MD Department of Cardiology,
University of Rochester Medical Center, Rochester,
NY, USA

Alon Barsheshet, MD Cardiology Department,
Rabin Medical Center, Petah Tiqva, Israel

Sackler Faculty of Medicine, Tel-Aviv University,
Tel-Aviv, Israel

Cardiology Division, University of Rochester Medical
Center, Rochester, New York

Andrew Brenyo, MD Arrhythmia Consultants, Greenville,
SC, USA

Ilan Goldenberg, MD Cardiology Department,
The Leviev Heart Center, Sheba Medical Center,
Tel Hashomer, Israel

Tel-Aviv University, Tel-Aviv, Israel

Cardiology Division, University of Rochester Medical
Center, Rochester, New York

Burr W. Hall, MD Department of Cardiology,
Atrial Fibrillation Clinic, University of Rochester
Medical Center, Rochester, NY, USA

David T. Huang, MD Department of Cardiology, University
of Rochester Medical Center, Rochester, NY, USA

Ryan Mandell, DO Department of Cardiology, University
of Rochester Medical Center, Rochester, NY, USA

Travis Prinzi, MD Department of Cardiology, University of Rochester Medical Center, Rochester, NY, USA

Spencer Rosero, MD Department of Cardiology, Hereditary Arrhythmia Clinic, University of Rochester Medical Center, Rochester, NY, USA

Sarah G. Taylor, MD Department of Cardiology, University of Rochester Medical Center, Rochester, NY, USA

Jeffrey M. Vinocur, MD Pediatric Electrophysiology Program, Golisano Children's Hospital, University of Rochester, Rochester, NY, USA

Chapter 1
Cardiac Conduction and Bradycardia

Mehmet K. Aktas and Ryan Mandell

Sinus Node, Atrioventricular Node, His-Purkinje System

The normal cardiac impulse originates from the sinoatrial (SA) node which is a small spindle shaped structure located anteriorly in the subepicardial region near the junction of the superior vena cava and the right atrium. The signal travels through the right atrium toward the left atrium and simultaneously inferiorly to the atrioventricular (AV) node (Figs. 1.1 and 1.2). The sinus node is innervated by both sympathetic and parasympathetic fibers that modulate the heart rate accordingly.

The AV node is located at the apex of the triangle of Koch, which is represented by the septal tricuspid valve annulus anteriorly, the coronary sinus ostium posteriorly, and the tendon of Todaro superiorly [1]. Acting as a gateway, the AV node exhibits decremental properties which help protect the ventricles from tachyarrhythmias starting from the atria. From here propagation continues inferiorly and anteriorly to

M.K. Aktas, MD (✉) • R. Mandell, DO
Department of Cardiology, University of Rochester Medical Center, Rochester, NY, USA
e-mail: mehmet_aktas@urmc.rochester.edu

D.T. Huang, T. Prinzi (eds.), *Clinical Cardiac Electrophysiology in Clinical Practice*, In Clinical Practice, DOI 10.1007/978-1-4471-5433-4_1, © Springer-Verlag London 2015

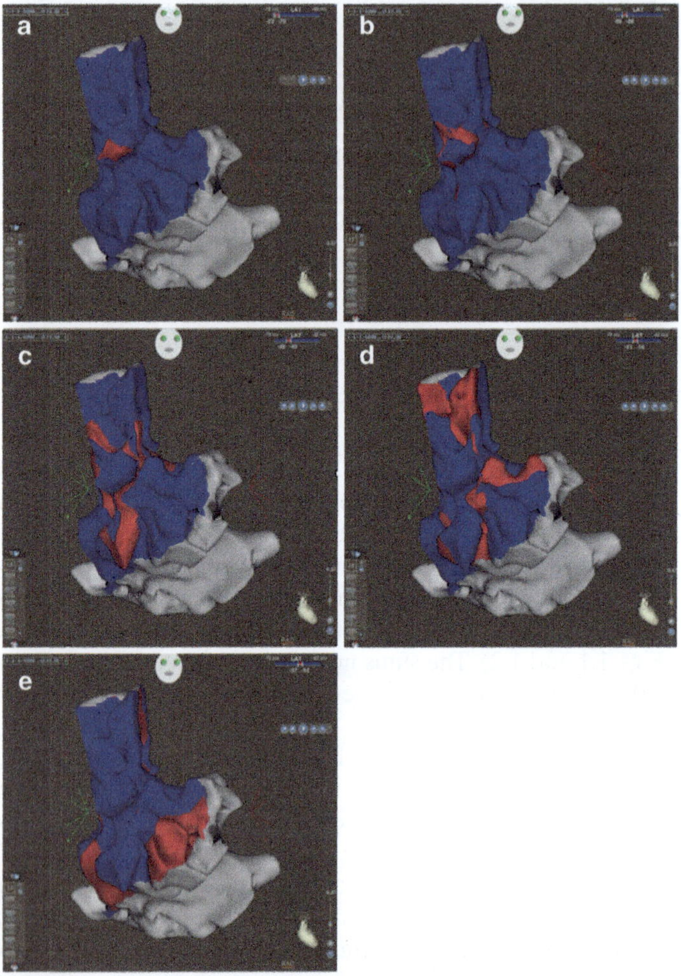

FIGURE 1.1 (**a–e**) Three dimensional reconstruction using CARTO (Biosense-Webster) of the RA showing sinus rhythm impulse propagation represented by the red wavefront as it spreads across the right atrium from the right anterior oblique view

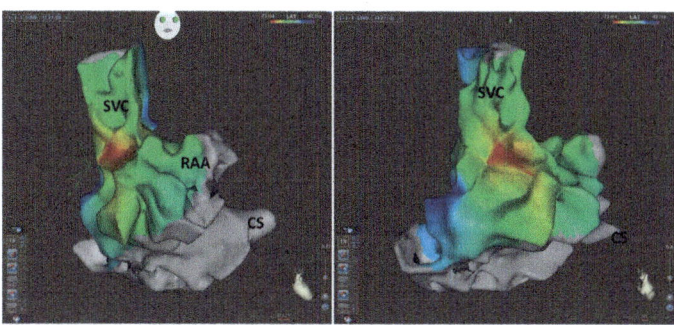

FIGURE 1.2 Three dimensional reconstruction using CARTO (Biosense-Webster) of the RA showing electroanatomical activation map showing site of origination of a sinus rhythm impulse, from the right anterior oblique (*left*) and right lateral (*right*) views. *Red* represents earliest activation and the sinus node's location. *Yellow, green, teal,* and *blue* represent respective later activation timing relative to the sinus node impulse. *SVC* superior vena cava, *CS* coronary sinus, *RAA* right atrial appendage

the bundle of His. Once the depolarizing wavefront exits the His bundle, the signal divides into three fascicles, the left anterior, the left posterior and the right bundle branch. Finally the impulse disseminates throughout the ventricular myocardium via smaller purkinje fibers. Conduction velocity is most rapid through the above activation sequence.

Patients may present in sinus rhythm with some clues to conduction disease on the surface ECG which may include either a prolonged PR interval, left anterior fascicular block (LAFB), left posterior fascicular block (LPFB), right bundle branch block (RBBB) or left bundle branch block (LBBB). Some patients may have more than one type of block such as first-degree AV block, fascicular block (either left anterior or left posterior) and RBBB. This combination is more commonly referred to trifascicular block. The remaining conduction to the ventricle is dependent on a single fascicle. In those patients with a left bundle branch block (both the left anterior and posterior fascicles are blocked) the conduction to the ventricle is through the right bundle. Usually the remaining bundle's conduction velocity is adequate to prevent symptoms, however, one should be more suspicious of a bradyarrhythmia as an etiology if multiple blocks are observed on the surface ECG. Of particular concern is alternating RBBB and LBBB as it is clear evidence of infra-nodal conduction disease. These patients should undergo pacemaker placement without the need for invasive electrophysiology testing as they are at high risk for complete heart block. Patients with bundle branch block particularly those with LBBB have been found to be at higher than normal risk for ventricular tachyarrhythmias and therefore it is important that such patients be thoroughly evaluated when presenting with syncope.

Each region of cardiac tissue is capable of generating an impulse (automaticity), however, the sinus node generally fires more rapidly and captures the remaining cardiac segments. A hierarchy of automaticity exists from the atria with a lower end rate limit of 40 bpm, to the AV node roughly 30–40 bpm, and the purkinje fibers 20–30 bpm. When there is impulse dysfunction in the atria the signal no longer suppresses the AV nodes automaticity and a junctional rhythm (usually narrow complex unless known bundle brach block) may be evident. If the rhythm originates from the purkinje fibers it is best described as an idioventricular rhythm, and will appear very slow with a wide QRS complex.

Sinus Node Dysfunction

Sinus node dysfunction is an umbrella term that refers to abnormalities in SN impulse formation and propagation and includes conditions such as sinus bradycardia, sinus pause/arrest, chronotropic incompetence, sinus exit block, sick sinus syndrome and tachy-brady syndrome where rapid periods of atrial fibrillation terminate often into symptomatic episodes of sinus bradycardia or sinus pauses. Sinus node dysfunction is a disease of the elderly and its initial presentation may include syncope due to inadequate impulse formation and propagation resulting in cerebral hypoperfusion and collapse [2]. Sinus node dysfunction is the most common diagnosis in patients requiring permanent pacemaker implant.

The action potentials of both the SA and AV node are dependent on sodium "funny" currents. These channels are recognized as funny because they open as the cell repolarizes rather than reaching a more positive threshold to evoke an action potential. The SA node traditionally depolarizes and repolarizes most rapidly and therefore is responsible for setting the heart rate if cardiac conduction is normal. Sympathetic (adrenaline) and parasympathetic (vagal) signals from the autonomic nervous system have strong influences on heart rate due to their primary inputs to the SA and AV node. Historically, a "normal" heart rate ranges from 60 to 100 beats per minute (bpm), however, it is not uncommon for those with high vagal tone (well conditioned athletes, or during sleep) to have rates as low as 40 bpm [3]. Electrocardiogram (ECG) tracings may reflect either a sinus bradycardia mechanism or a junctional escape rhythm (an impulse originating from the AV node.) Bradycardia in and of itself is not problematic unless it is associated with symptoms such as dizziness, fatigue, shortness of breath, chest pain or syncope [4]. On the contrary, patient's may present with exertional symptoms despite resting heart rates in the 60s. Placing these patients on a treadmill or on a Holter monitor may reveal chronotropic incompetence, or lack of the SA node to increase the heart rate appropriately with activity [5]. It is important to make the distinction between physiologic bradycardia and symptomatic pathologic bradycardia to avoid unnecessary testing or treatments which may only cause harm and or provide little to no benefit. Furthermore, the etiology of the arrhythmia must strongly be considered. Electrolyte imbalance, ischemia, infection, hypoxia, vagal tone, hypothermia, hypothyroidism, post surgical as well as other causes may be transient and treating the underlying cause may very well resolve the cardiac conduction disturbance [6, 7]. Temporary pacemakers may be considered in specific emergent situations as deemed necessary.

Atrioventricular Block

AV block can be classified as first, second or third degree (also known as complete heart block). Although a distinct conduction fiber between the sinus node and this His-bundle does not exist, first degree AV block refers to a PR interval exceeding 0.2 s. A long PR interval in the setting of a normal QRS duration usually represents conduction delay in the AV node. If the QRS duration is prolonged, the most common site of conduction delay is still in the AV node, however the possibility of infra-Hisian conduction disease needs to be considered, especially in the presence of left bundle branch block. It is important however to recognize that a normal PR interval does not itself rule out the possibility of more advanced and severe conduction disease. In general, first degree AV block is clinically well tolerated and is not associated with an increase in overall mortality. However, in rare cases a PR exceeding 0.3 s can produce pacemaker syndrome-like symptoms where atrial activation begins as ventricular systole continues, and atrial contraction occurs across closed atrio-ventricular valves.

Second degree AV block (Fig. 1.3) is subdivided into Mobitz Type 1 and Mobitz Type 2 block.

Electrocardiographically, Mobitz type 1 exhibits the Wenckebach phenomenon where progressive prolongation in the PR interval is seen leading up to a non-conducted P wave. Following the non-conducted beat, conduction with a normal PR interval is usually seen. The block cycle recurs repetitively with a fixed P to QRS ratio. Most commonly AV block in Mobitz 1 occurs at the level of the AV node less so in the His-Purkinje system. Mobitz Type 1 block is common in healthy individuals and in states of high vagal innervation such as during sleep. However, Mobitz Type 1 block that occurs during high sympathetic innervation such as with exercise usually denotes infra-Hisian disease possibly requiring electrophysiologic testing [8]. Contrary, Mobitz Type 2 block demonstrates a fixed PR interval with a non-conducted P wave. Maneuvers like carotid sinus

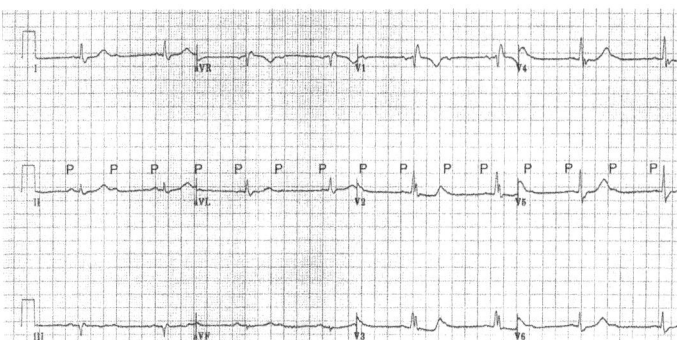

FIGURE 1.3 12 lead electrocardiogram demonstrating 2:1 AV block. There are 2 p waves for every qrs complex. It is not possible to tell where the level of block is without provocative maneuvers such as having the patient ambulate, vagal maneuvers or administering medications which can inhibit or enhance AV node conduction

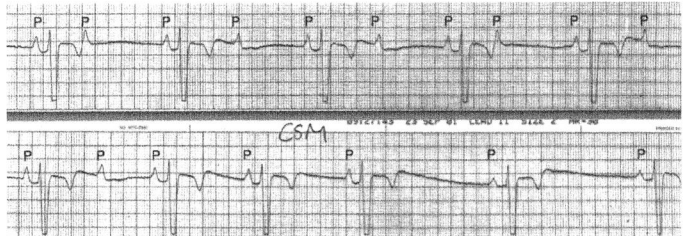

FIGURE 1.4 2:1 AV block is present throughout the top telemetry strip. During carotid sinus massage (CSM) the increased vagal tone creates a 1:1 AV relationship. This is indicative of infranodal disease and best treated with a permanent pacemaker

massage can be useful for differentiating between Mobtiz Type 1 and Type 2 block when there is 2:1 conduction. For Mobitz Type 1 block the higher vagal input to the AV node will increase the amount of blocked p waves. However, for Mobitz Type 2 block the higher vagal input to the AV node will slow conduction enough to let the diseased infrahisian tissue time to recover allowing for a 1:1 relationship (Fig. 1.4).

Complete heart block is present when atrial activation does not conduct to the ventricles. Complete heart block may occur as a result of pathology within the AV node or in infranodal conducting fibers. In patients with complete heart block often an escape rhythm is present, either a narrow complex junctional rhythm or a wide complex ventricular rhythm. Patients with complete heart block may present with dizziness, presyncope and syncope. Patients with complete heart are also at risk for ventricular tachycardia and ventricular fibrillation.

Electrophysiologic Testing

Occasionally, it may be difficult to correlate if a patient's symptoms are related to a bradyarrhythmia through noninvasive testing, and an electrophysiology study (EPS) may be required. An EPS allows for an objective measurement of the cardiac conduction system. Catheters are placed into the heart to evaluate for dysfunction of either impulse formation or propagation. A catheter is usually placed in the right atrium, the coronary sinus, near the bundle of His, and into the right ventricle. The catheters have the ability to both sense electrical potentials as well as pace. Spanning the catheters into each of the locations facilitate accurate diagnosis and location of potential conduction disease. Baseline measurements which are noted on the surface ECG are recorded including the PR interval, QRS duration and QT interval. On the intracardiac electrocardiograms, the PR interval is reflected by the activation from the A (atria) to the H (His bundle) and the V (ventricular) signal. Of particular importance is the assessment of the HV interval. A measurement greater than 100 ms is highly abnormal and warrants pacemaker placement [2]. First degree AV block, better characterized as AV delay, is reflected in prolongation of the AH interval with normal conduction once the His bundle is activated.

Second degree heart block Mobitz Type 1 or Wenkebach is demonstrated by continued prolongation of the AH interval until there is loss of His bundle activation due to block occurring in the AV node. This type of block is considered physiological and not pathologic. In fact, Wenckebach is commonly observed during an EP study due to the decremental properties of the AV node.

Second degree heart block type two arises when the AH interval is constant and the block occurs inferior to the His bundle. This is considered abnormal and is concerning for risk of progression into third degree or complete heart block. Complete heart block is evident based on no corresponding relationship between the atria and ventricles. Isorhythmic dissociation may make the diagnosis of complete heart block more difficult as both the atria and ventricles are conducting at the same rate. Pacing the atria at a faster rate with intracardiac catheters can help make this distinction or a beta agonist can accelerate the atrial rate revealing the atria and ventricle were coincidently at the same rate and that they are truly dissociated.

Pacing maneuvers during EPS will provide an objective measurement of the sinus and AV node (both antegrade and retrograde) function. Sinus node recovery time (SNRT) is measured by pacing to atrium at 30 s faster than the intrinsic sinus rate to suppress sinus node automaticity. The recovery time is measured from the last pacing stimuli to the onset of sinus node activity on the intra cardiac electrocardiogram. Less than 1,500 milliseconds (ms) is considered normal or less than 550 ms for the corrected SNRT (sinus cycle length in msec minus the SNRT). Patients may also demonstrate sinus node exit block where an electrical impulse is unable to penetrate through the perinodal tissue due to prolonged refractory periods. This may occur either as a Mobitz one or two block. One may see a sinus rate at 600 ms and then the absence of a p wave at half the interval between the two conducted p waves. The remainder of the sinus rhythm will be consistent at 600 ms.

One can then assess the functional properties of the AV node via pacing stimuli including the cycle length at which Wenckebach occurs or when atrial activation blocks in the AV node and does not conduct into the His bundle. If the block occurs after His activation then Mobitz type two block is present which is important distinction from Wenckebach (Fig. 1.5). Wenckebach will show AH interval prolongation on the His catheter as the cycle length is decreased in a stepwise fashion by 10 ms. This is traditionally done with a pacing train which is several beats at a given rate prior to the last beat which is 10 ms less then the last beat in the prior pacing train. For example, eight beats at 600 ms followed by a 500 ms beat. Then eight beats at 600 ms followed by a 490 ms beat. A stepwise approach will assess for dual AV nodal physiology or a 10 ms decrease in cycle length will demonstrate AH prolongation by 50 ms suggesting block down the fast pathway and activation of the His bundle through an additional AV nodal slow pathway. A thorough EPS will help rule out all potential arrhythmogenic etiologies for a patient's clinical presentation. Ventricular pacing can assess the presence of VA or retrograde conduction (Fig. 1.6). Activation should be concentric on the CS catheter or activating from proximally to distally. An eccentric activation sequence can suggest an accessory pathway that may only conduct retrogradely and therefore would not show any pre-excitation. Para-hisian pacing or near the His bundle can help exclude a paraseptal pathway. The electrical output is maximized to capture the His bundle which generates a narrow QRS. The output is gradually decreased. An AV nodal response is lack of direct His capture leading to a wide QRS as well as prolonged VA time if present. If the QRS remains narrow even at low outputs a paraseptal accessory pathway is most likely present. Understanding the normal functioning properties of the AV node is essential to help exclude the potential for either brady- or tachyarrhythmias.

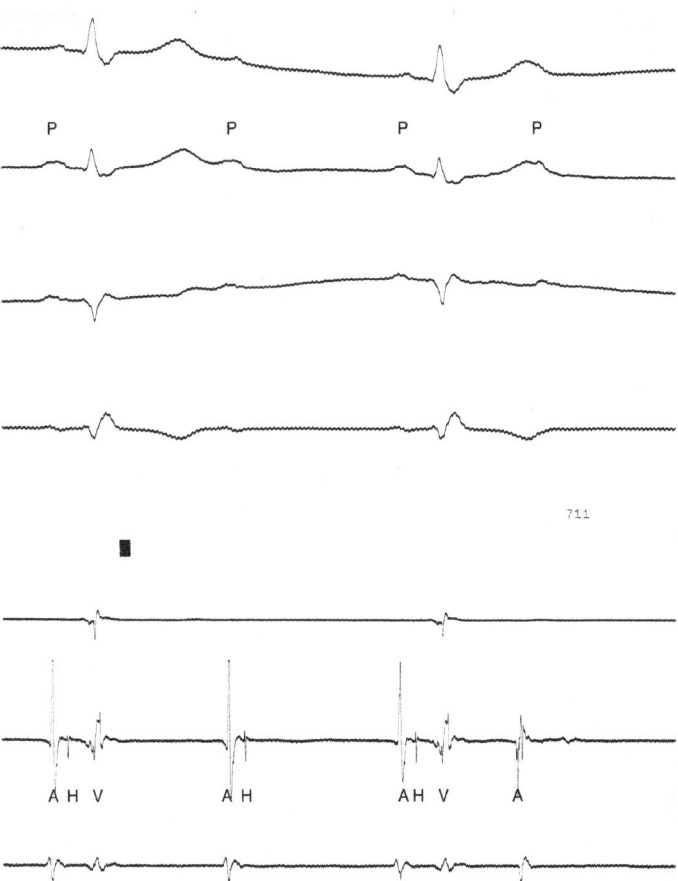

FIGURE 1.5 The first sinus beat conducts through the AV node with subsequent activation of the His bundle followed by ventricular activation. The second sinus beat conducts through the AV node to the His bundle and blocks below the His. The 3rd sinus beat conducts similar to the first beat since the infrahisian level of block had time to recover from the prior blocked beat. The last beat is a premature atrial contraction and blocks in the AV node as there is no His activation. The second beat is considered pathological and warrants placement of a pacemaker. *P* atrial activation on the surface electrocardiogram, *A* atrial activation on the intracardiac electrogram, *H* His bundle activation on the intracardiac electrogram, *V* ventricular activation on the intracardiac electrogram

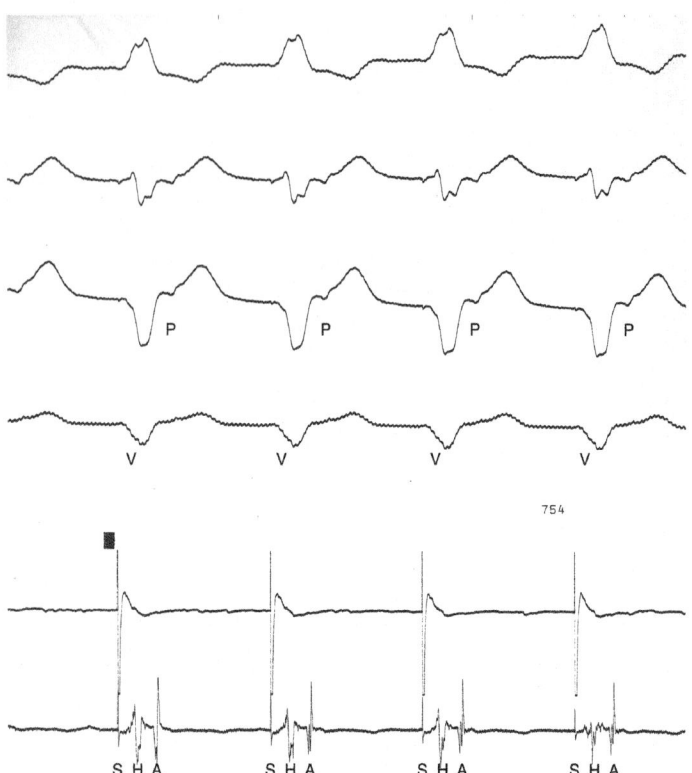

754

FIGURE 1.6 Ventricular pacing demonstrating intact retrograde ventricular-atrial conduction with activation of a His potential prior to atrial activation during an EPS. *V* ventricular activation on surface electrocardiogram, *P* inverted p wave consistent with retrograde conduction from ventricular pacing, *S* pacing stimulation artifact from right ventricular catheter, *H* His bundle activation on the intracardiac electrogram, *A* atrial electrogram on the intracardiac electrogram which coincides with the P wave on the surface electrocardiogram

Concealed Conduction and Incomplete Impulse Penetration

Concealed conduction refers to incomplete impulse penetration into the normal AV nodal conduction system producing ECG findings that could otherwise not be explained, hence the term concealed conduction. Antegrade as well as retrograde concealed conduction into the normal AV nodal conduction system may occur. A common site of retrograde concealment is when a PVC conducts retrogradely into the His-Purkinje system causing antegrade AV block of the following sinus beat. Another common circumstance where concealed conduction is observed is in the development and continuation of aberrant conduction during supraventricular tachycardias.

Gap Phenomenon

A gap in AV conduction is observed when AV conduction block is observed with a premature atrial beat, but a subsequent atrial beat of greater prematurity successfully conducts to the ventricles. The Gap phenomenon occurs as a result of functional differences in conduction present in different regions of the conduction system, often requiring a distal segment with a long refractory period and proximal segment with a shorter refractory period. As such, a premature beat conducts successfully to the distal segment where block occurs. However, with increasing prematurity the beat encounters delayed conduction in the proximal segment giving the distal segment time to recover thereby allowing conduction.

Transient Bundle Branch Block

Intermittent bundle branch block can be due to several different mechanisms. In phase 3 block, aberrancy results from encroachment of the impulse on the refractory period of the tissue the impulse is conducting through. Rate dependent transient bundle branch block occurs when a critical heart rate is reached. Phase 4 block, also known as bradycardia dependent block, occurs in diseased His-Purkinje system where a loss in the resting membrane potential is observed. Finally, as mentioned above, retrograde concealment into a bundle branch may result in transient bundle branch block.

Congenital Heart Block

Newborns may present with conduction disease spanning from first degree block to complete heart block. Children from mother's who have systemic lupus erythematosus are at higher risk of acquiring complete heart block. Antibodies cross the placenta during utero and evoke an immune response that leads to scarring and fibrosis around the AV node [9]. Some patients may have congenital cardiac structural anomalies which may require surgery. In these instances patients may acquire cardiac conduction disease due to post surgical changes. Consideration of a permanent pacemaker will depend on the underlying escape mechanism's rate, and the patient's symptoms.

Neuromuscular Diseases

Clinicians need to be aware of several neuromuscular conditions which are associated with AV block. Common neuromuscular conditions that are associated with cardiac conduction disease include progressive familial heart block, facioscapulohumeral syndrome, myotonic dystrophy, Kearns-Sayre Syndrome, Fredreich's ataxia, and Erb's dystrophy [10–12]. Progression from normal conduction to high degree AV block may occur rapidly and unpredictably in such patients and therefore close surveillance is recommended.

References

1. Spragg DD, Tomaselli GF. Chapter 232. The bradyarrhythmias. In: Longo DL, Fauci AS, Kasper DL, Hauser SL, Jameson J, Loscalzo J, editors. Harrison's principles of internal medicine. 18th ed. New York: McGraw-Hill; 2012.
2. Epstein AE, et al. ACC/AHA/HRS 2008 guidelines for device-based therapy of cardiac rhythm abnormalities. Heart Rhythm. 2008;5(6):934–55.
3. Talan DA, Bauernfeind RA, et al. Twenty-four hour continuous ECG recordings in long-distance runners. Chest. 1982;82(1):19–24.
4. Ferrer MI. The sick sinus syndrome in atrial disease. JAMA. 1968;206(3):645–6.
5. Katritsis D, Camm AJ. Chronotropic incompetence: a proposal for definition and diagnosis. Br Heart J. 1993;70:400–2.
6. Grimm W, Koehler U, et al. Outcome of patients with sleep apnea-associated severe bradyarrhythmias after continuous positive airway pressure therapy. Am J Cardiol. 2000;86:688–92, A9.
7. Kim MH, Deeb GM, et al. Complete atrioventricular block after valvular heart surgery and the timing of pacemaker implantation. Am J Cardiol. 2001;87:649–51, A10.
8. Dhingra RC, Denes P, et al. The significance of second degree atrioventricular block and bundle branch block. Observations regarding site and type of block. Circulation. 1974;49(4):638–46.
9. Cunningham F, Leveno KJ, Bloom SL, Hauth JC, Rouse DJ, Spong CY. Chapter 29. Diseases and injuries of the fetus and newborn. In: Cunningham F, Leveno KJ, Bloom SL, Hauth JC, Rouse DJ, Spong CY, editors. Williams obstetrics. 23rd ed. New York: McGraw-Hill; 2010.
10. Hiromasa S, Ikeda T, et al. Myotonic dystrophy: ambulatory electrocardiogram, electrophysiologic study, and echocardiographic evaluation. Am Heart J. 1987;113:1482–8.
11. Stevenson WG, Perloff JK, et al. Facioscapulohumeral muscular dystrophy: evidence for selective, genetic electrophysiologic cardiac involvement. J Am Coll Cardiol. 1990;15:292–9.
12. James TN, Fisch C. Observations on the cardiovascular involvement in Friedreich's ataxia. Am Heart J. 1963;66:164–75.

Chapter 2
Syncope, Tilt Testing, and Cardioversion

Sarah G. Taylor

Syncope is a diagnostic and therapeutic challenge affecting an impressive number of patients. Syncope accounts for 3 % of emergency room visit and 6 % of all hospital admissions [22]. The lifetime incidence of syncope is close to 40 % [7]. Syncope has a bimodal distribution of occurrence, the prevalence is high between 10 and 30 years, not a common occurrence in middle life, and then peaks again after the age of 65 [16] (Fig. 2.1).

One of the most interested yet challenging features regarding the management of syncope is the diverse range of significance of a syncopal episode. Syncope can be a very benign, explicable almost anticipated outcome of a predictable setting. On the other hand, syncope may the one and only presenting symptom of a life threatening disease. Given the staggeringly broad causes and consequences of a syncopal episode, the treating physician has two goals.

S.G. Taylor, MD
Department of Cardiology, University of Rochester Medical Center, Rochester, NY, USA
e-mail: sarah_taylor@urmc.rochester.edu

D.T. Huang, T. Prinzi (eds.), *Clinical Cardiac Electrophysiology in Clinical Practice*, In Clinical Practice, DOI 10.1007/978-1-4471-5433-4_2,
© Springer-Verlag London 2015

Age of first faint

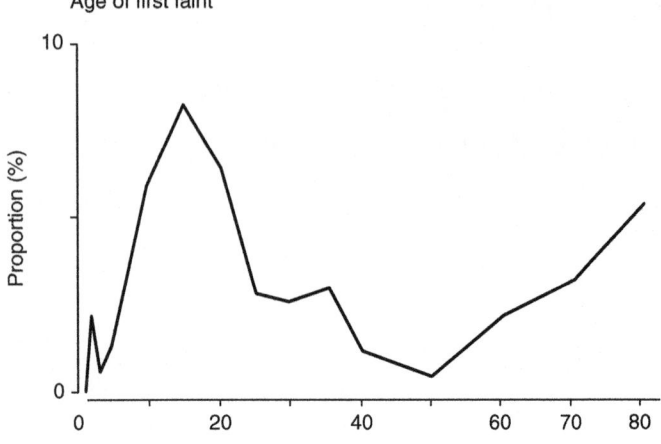

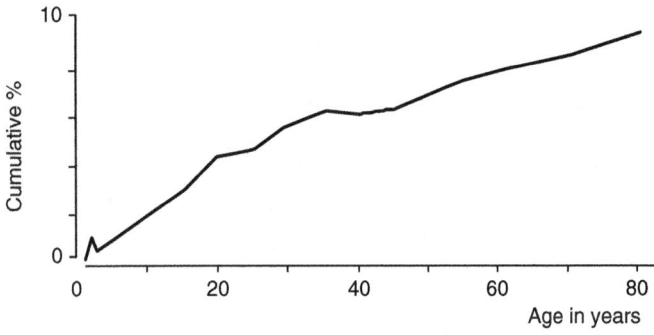

Age in years

FIGURE 2.1 Age in years

1. Identify the cause of the syncope in order to guide treatment based on the underlying etiology
2. Identify the specific risk to the patient. This includes not only the risk of recurrent syncope, but also the risks associated with the underlying [16].

For the physician managing syncope, risk stratification, which is based on the etiology of the syncopal episode, becomes perhaps the most important role.

Syncope is derived from the Greek word synkopē, which means "to cut short" or "to interrupt". Syncope is defined by

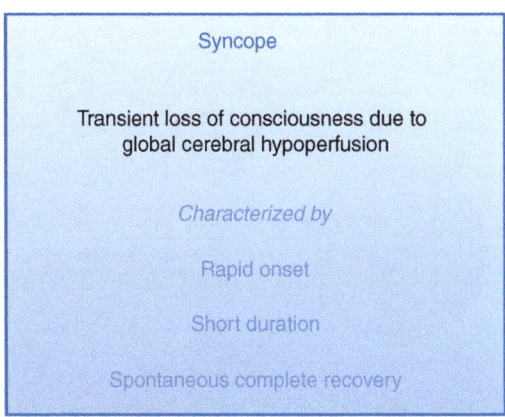

FIGURE 2.2 Syncope Defined

transient loss of consciousness due to global cerebral hypo-perfusion. Syncope is characterized by rapid onset, short duration, and spontaneous complete recovery.

There are many syndromes that may present as masquerading syncope. These include falls, cataplexy, TIAs, seizures, psychogenic pseudosyncope, metabolic disorders, intoxication, and vertebrobasilar insufficiency. Because of confusion in the etiology of these episodes, many of these patients are referred to the electrophysiologist for the evaluation of the cardiac conduction system. It is important to discern the features that suggest a non-syncopal alternation in consciousness. A thorough history should differentiate these other forms of altered consciousness from the sudden loss of consciousness due to a global, reversible reduction in blood flow (Fig. 2.2).

Testing done in the electrophysiology lab is performed to evaluate whether syncope resulted from bradycardia, tachycardia, or a reproducible cardiac reflex or autonomic abnormality. Prior to undergoing testing, a thorough history is essential to help correctly classify syncope. The 2009 European Society of Cardiology guidelines for the management of syncope provide an excellent framework for the classification of syncope based on etiology [3] (Fig. 2.3).

Insufficient cerebral perfusion is the hallmark of syncope. The insults that result in an abrupt reduction of cerebral

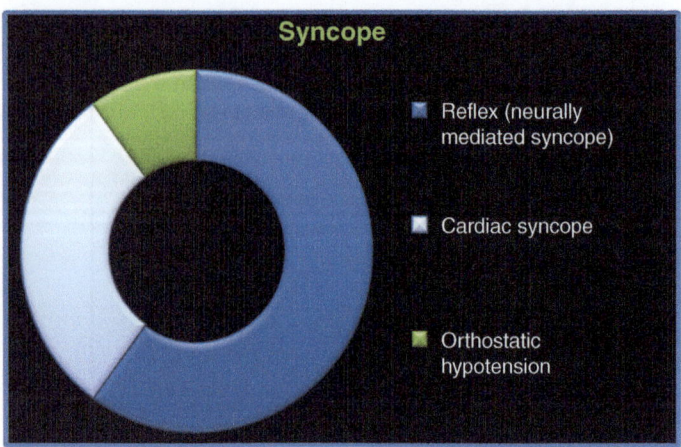

Figure 2.3 Relative incidence of syncope by pathophysiological classification

blood flow are many and varied. A fall in systemic blood pressure curtails global cerebral blood flow. If blood flow is significant diminished for as short as for 6–8 s, syncope may ensue. Systemic blood pressure is determined by systemic vascular resistance and cardiac output. Cardiac output is the product of heart rate and stroke volume. Syncope may result from a decrease in peripheral vascular resistance, a reduction in heart rate, a reduction in stroke volume, or a reduction in a combination of mechanisms [16] (Fig. 2.4).

Reflex Syncope

Reflex syncope, also correctly termed neutrally mediated syncope, accounts for more than half of syncope. Determining the mechanism of the reflex syncope episodes is paramount for effective treatment and prevention. Reflex syncope should be thought of as a spectrum of inappropriate reflexes. Vasodepressor syncope, characterized by a profound hypotensive response is at one end of the spectrum and cardioinhibitory syncope, characterized by asystolic pauses, is at the other end of the spectrum. While the etiology is the same, the

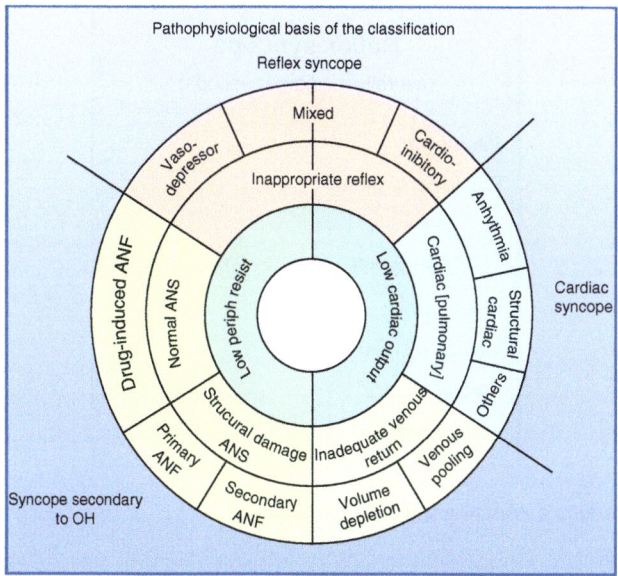

FIGURE 2.4 Pathophysiologic Basis of the Classification of Syncope

hemodynamic responses may be markedly different. Identifying where on this spectrum the patient lies, guides the treating physician to effective therapy. No longer is it appropriate to apply across the board treatment to the spectrum of neutrally mediated syncope. For patients in whom a vasodepressor response is the overriding perturbation, volume expansion, vasoconstriction and blood pressure augmentation is the mainstay of treatment. Patients that have a primary cardioinhibitory response to reflex-provoking stimuli may benefit from pacemaker therapy. This has been demonstrated in the Eastbourne Syncope Assessment Study, where implantable loop recorders effectively guided syncope therapy [6].

The most common etiology of syncope is a neutrally mediated reflex triggered by different stimuli leading to sudden withdrawal of sympathetic activity and to an increase in parasympathetic nerve tone. The results are vasodilatation and bradycardia. Neurally mediated syncope is classically precipitated extrinsic factors, be it physical or emotional triggers.

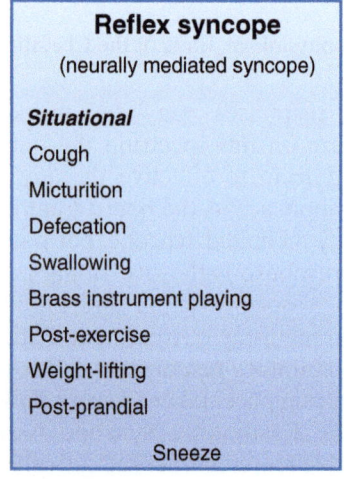

Reflex syncope

(neurally mediated syncope)

Vasovagal

Emotional triggers

Fear

Orthostatic stress

Phlebotomy

Medical instrumentation

Trauma

Stage Fright

FIGURE 2.5 Vasovagal Reflex Syncope

Reflex syncope

(neurally mediated syncope)

Situational

Cough

Micturition

Defecation

Swallowing

Brass instrument playing

Post-exercise

Weight-lifting

Post-prandial

Sneeze

FIGURE 2.6 Situational Reflex Syncope

This includes prolonged standing leading to venous pooling as well as emotional triggers such as fear, needle phobia, pain, and stage fright (Fig. 2.5).

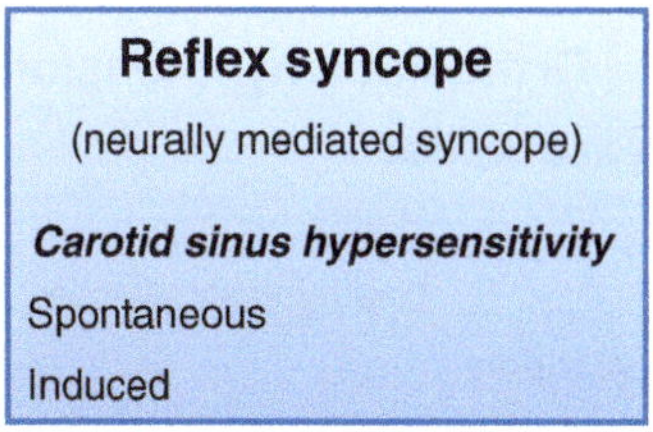

Reflex syncope

(neurally mediated syncope)

Carotid sinus hypersensitivity

Spontaneous

Induced

FIGURE 2.7 Carotid Sinus Hypersensitiity Reflex Syncope

Another form of neutrally mediated syncope is situational syncope. There are specific triggers that elicit abnormal hemodynamic responses leading to the symptomatic global hypoperfusion (Fig. 2.6).

Carotid sinus hypersensitivity is another form of reflex syncope. While other forms of reflex syncope may occurs throughout all stages of life, this typically presents >50 years of age. It is more common in men than in women. An abnormal response to carotid sinus massage is defined as a pause for more than three seconds or a drop in systolic blood pressure greater than 50 mmHg. Normally a mixed picture of vasodepressor and cardioinhibitory response is elicited (Fig. 2.7).

Syncope Due to Orthostatic Hypotension

An abnormal vasoconstriction response to upright position can results in decreased cerebral perfusion. When upright, 10–15 % of blood pools in the lower extremities. The baroreceptors are activated by the decreased pressure that results from this drop in venous return and drop in stroke volume. A normal response increased heart rate, increased contractility and restored vascular tone. However, an abnormal response to these triggers may result in orthostatic intolerance if normal stroke volume is not restored. An abnormal response to upright posture is defined as a decrease in systolic blood pressure >20 mmHg or a decrease of symptomatic fall of systolic blood pressure associated with syncope or pre-syncope (Fig. 2.8).

Orthostatic hypotension

Volume depletion

> Hemorrhage
>
> Gastrointestinallosses

Medication

> Vasodilators
>
> Alpha–blockers

Diurtics

Neuromodulators

Primary autonomic failure

> Multiple–system atrophy
>
> Parkinson's
>
> Pure autonomic failure

Secondary autonomic failure

> Diabetes
>
> Amyloidosis
>
> Uremia
>
> Spinal cord injuries

Figure 2.8 Orthostatic Hypotension Syncope

Cardiac Syncope

Cardiac syncope requires the most accurate diagnosis, as it may be the first sign of a life-threatening disorder. The absence of a prodrome is a common feature of these high-risk syncope scenarios. As a result, the risk of trauma is much higher with cardiac syncope. Exertional syncope should initiate a search for a cardiac cause of syncope (Figs. 2.9 and 2.10).

Obstruction to cardiac output is another cause of syncope. While this type of cardiac syncope is less common, it carries with it a high mortality [17].

Arrhythmias also impede cardiac output. The sudden change in heart rate, wither fast or slow, may drastically reduce the cardiac output. In some patients with SVT, the

Cardiac syncope

Tachyarrhythmia

Supraventricular tachycardia

A trial fibrillation

A VNRT

A VRT

Wolff-Parkinson white

syndrome

Ventricular tachyarrhythmias

Long QT syndrome

Ischemia

Hypertrophic cardiomyopathy

ARVD

Short QT syndrome

Brugada syndrome

CPVT

Cardiac sarcoidosis

Drugs

Idiopathic VF

Left ventricular dysfunnction

Bradyarrhythmia

Sinus node arrest

Sinoatrial block

A V block

Infrahisian conduction diseae
pacemarker or ICD malfunction

Structural heart abnormalities

Aortic stenosis

Hypertrophic cardiomyopathy

Mitral stenosis

A trial myxoma

Pericardial tamponade

Pulmonary hypertenasion

Pulmonary embolism

Myocardialischemia or infarction

FIGURE 2.9 Cardiac Syncope

> *"The only difference between syncope and sudden death is that in one you wake up"* –George Engel

Figure 2.10

cardiac output is still sufficient to maintain cerebral perfusion, but a mixed picture with a vasodepressor response occurs, resulting in syncope [12].

In patient with a suspicion for arrhythmogenic syncope, but yet undocumented rhythm disturbances, lengthy monitoring is often required. The implantable loop recorder has proven to be very useful in this regard. The ILR provides a cost-efficient and timely method to correlate heart rhythm at the time of syncope or presyncopal symptoms. This leads to the appropriate intervention, be it pacemaker, defibrillator, electrophysiology study with ablation, or medical therapy. Even documenting normal sinus rhythm at the time of symptoms can efficiently reroute the management in the effective direction (Fig. 2.11).

Tilt Table Testing

Tilt table testing is utilized to help investigate the underlying cause of unexplained syncope. Tilt table testing was first used to diagnose syncope in 1986 [10]. The test helps demonstrate the hemodynamic response to a passive upright challenge. It can help define the mechanism with neutrally mediated syncope or orthostatic hypotension syncope is suspected. If the detailed clinical history, along with a normal exam, normal echo, and normal ECG all suggest neutrally mediated syncope, a tilt table test may not be necessary to solidify the diagnosis [5]. However, there are times when a formal test is useful. Fortunately, tilt table testing is easy, safe, well tolerated, and often contributes to the patients understanding of

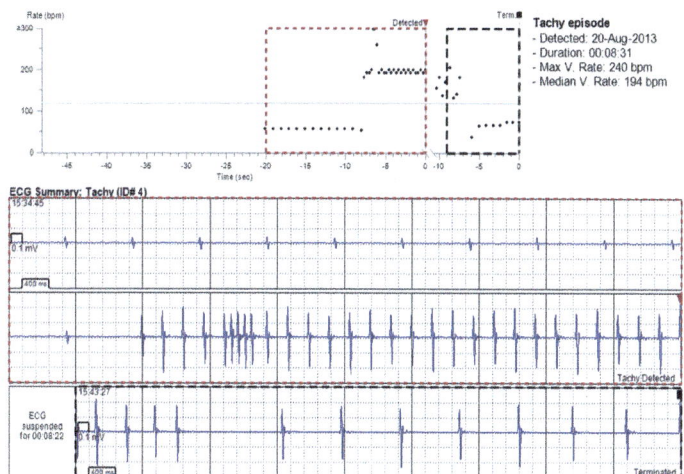

FIGURE 2.11 Medtronic Carelink Event Monitor Sample Report [25]

their clinical situation. It also plays a role in defining dysautonomia syndromes, such as postural orthostatic tachycardia syndrome and orthostatic intolerance.

Tilt table testing is also utilized to diagnose pseudosyncope, recurrent falls, and occasionally for medication guidance. Tilt table testing has been useful for initiating and monitoring pyridostigmine therapy. Tilt table testing with EEG can be useful for differentiating seizures from syncope, as well as for diagnosed pseudoseizures or pseudosyncope (Fig. 2.12).

Tilt table testing can be performed safely at all ages [8, 11, 23]. Well operating equipment is paramount. Attentive staff with continuous hemodynamic monitoring is required. The tilt must be able to be reliably and quickly reversed. While there are rare reports of arrhythmias and myocardial infarction during tilt table testing, these risks are typically related to the provocation. There are no reports of death from tilt table testing.

Ideally, tilt table testing should be carried out in a room free of distractions and overstimulation. The environment

Contraindications for tilt testing

Inability to cooperate

Pregnancy

Critical valvular stenosis

LVOT obstruction

Severe proximal cerebral stenosis

Severe coronary artery disease

Recent MI

Recent CVA

Weight that exceeds safe table operation

FIGURE 2.12   Contraindication to Tilt Testing

should be at a constant temperature, avoiding excessing heat or cold to avoid autonomic triggers. The test should be observed continuously as restoring the patient to the supine position is integral to restoring cerebral perfusion.

Protocols to improve the sensitivity of the tilt table test include using provocative agents [18]. Isoproterenol infusions have been used. Nitroglycerin is a provocative agent that is better tolerated, especially in elderly patients [24]. The "Italian Protocol" for upright tilt test involves a stabilization phase of 5 min in the supine position, passive tilt phase of 20 min at a tilt angle of 60°; and provocation phase of further 15 min of 60° tilt after sublingual nitroglycerin.. Carotid sinus massage during tilt can also increase the diagnostic yield of testing for carotid sinus hypersensitivity [15]. Care must be taken to weigh the risk of stroke during carotid massage, as the risk is approximately 1:1,000 [19].

The test should be completed to the end of protocol. Test interruption is made when the protocol is completed in the absence of symptoms, or there is occurrence of syncope, or occurrence of progressive (>5 min) orthostatic hypotension [2]. Transient asystole, and at times prolonged asystole, may be precipitated. Rarely are interventions other than returning to supine are required (Fig. 2.13).

Reasons for early termination of tilt table testing

Sycncope

Systolic BP < 70 mmHg or rapid decline

Bradycardia < 50 bpm or rapid decline

Execssive tachycardia (exceeding 220-age)

Significant arrhytnmias

Hyperventilation leading to $ETCO_2 < 20$ mmHg

Patient distress

Unstable patient positioning

FIGURE 2.13 Termination of Tilt Testing

Interpreting the Results

A positive tilt table test demonstrates an abnormal hemodynamic response to upright challenge with the symptom reproduction. When a patient's syncope or presyncope symptoms are reproduced and accompanied by bradycardia and hypotension, a diagnosis of neutrally mediated syncope is suspected. The degree of relative bradycardia versus hypotension can help elucidate cardioinhibitory versus vasodepressor syncope. When hemodynamic changes occur in the absence of symptoms, the test is deemed a false positive. Clearly, a limiting feature of tilt table test is the false positive response to the test. The test must be interpreted in the context of the clinical scenario (Fig. 2.14).

Cardioversion

Perhaps the simplest yet most utilized and useful tool in cardiac electrophysiology is the cardioversion. It is also the most historical application of electricity. In fact an animal application in poultry to induce and correct arrhythmias was documented in the eighteenth century [1]. Karl Ludwig applied electrical current to a canine heart in 1850 [20]. The first human intentional application was in 1947 using DC defibril-

Hemodynamic response to upright tilt test

Postural orthostatic tachycardia syndrome

Heart rate exceeds > 130 bpm in the first 10 min of upright challenge. Significant hypotension is not part of the typical response.

Vasodepressor

Decline in blood pressure with the absence of herat rate decline > 10 %

CardioInhibitory

Heart rate drops to < 40 pm

Asystolic response

Mixed hemodynamic response

Bradycardia with hypotension

Orthostatic hypotension

Sustained fall in systolic blood pressure > 20 mmHG or diastolic blood pressure > 10 mmHg in the first 3 min of tilt

FIGURE 2.14 Hemodynamic responses to Upright Tilt Testing

lation during cardiac surgery. The first application of cardioversion to convert atrial fibrillation was in 1962. Lown utilized synchronized DC shocks to restore normal sinus rhythm [13, 14].

More recent improvements in the technique of cardioversion include using defibrillation electrodes or pads that adhere to the patient's skin rather than using paddles. Another advancement that has improved the efficacy of energy delivery to the heart while minimizing concurrent myocardial damage is the use of biphasic rather than monophasic waveforms.

Prior to cardioversion, electrolytes should be evaluated and corrected if abnormal. If necessary, digoxin levels should be evaluated and acute myocardial infarction excluded. Anticoagulation should be administered prior to cardioversion. Documentation of adequate uninterrupted anticoagulation in the weeks prior to cardioversion is necessary to minimize the risk of cardioembolic phenomenon. If adequate anticoagulation cannot be ensured, TEE-guided cardioversion should be employed. While traditionally the duration of AF that mandated anticoagulation was thought to be 48 h, there is increasing data suggesting that the risk of stroke may be associated with much shorter episodes of AF [9, 21].

Adequate monitored anesthesia care or monitored sedation is a critical part of cardioversion. Patient comfort in this elective procedure is paramount. Synchronization of the electrical discharge with the QRS complex is what differentiates cardioversion from defibrillation. By timing the electrical discharge with the QRS, the vulnerable period of the T wave is avoided. The risk of inducing ventricular fibrillation exists is a shock was delivered during this vulnerable window. Defibrillation is an unsynchronized delivery of energy used to convert ventricular fibrillation. Care should be taken not to try to synchronize the defibrillation to a rhythm of ventricular fibrillation as delays in therapy may occur. When an electrical current delivered across the myocardium, the cells are simultaneously depolarized, reset, and permit restoration of sinus node activation. The sinus node takes over as the effective pacemaker. Cardioversion is effective for the termination of atrial fibrillation, ventricular tachycardia, or reentrant SVTs. Some arrhythmias will not terminate with cardioversion, notably arrhythmias due to increased automaticity. This includes digitalis-induced tachycardia, catecholamine induced arrhythmia, and some focal atrial tachycardias.

Once the electrodes and defibrillation pads are applies, the defibrillator should be synchronized to detect the patients R waves. When adequately sedated, the energy level is selected and the shock button is pressed and held until discharge. There is a momentarily delay until the defibrillator discharges with the next detected R wave, thereby avoiding delivering energy in the vulnerable period of the cardiac cycle [26] (Fig. 2.15).

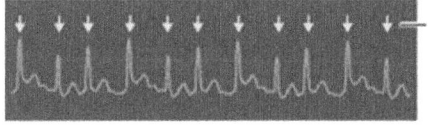

Marker indicates each detected R wave during synchronization

FIGURE 2.15 Synchronizing to R Waves

Guide for successful cardioversion

Adequate skin preparation

Dry, clean, and hairless

Optimal electrode placement for optimal current flow

> AP placement is preferable

> Anterior pad should be on the right lateral border of the sternum centered over the fourth intercostal space

> Posterior pad should be placed adjacent to the left of the spine with the center of the electrode at the level of the T7 vertabra

No air pockets or uneven adhesion of pads

Appropiate selection of energy

> For atrial flutter, energy levels between 30–100 J biphasic will be effective

> For atrial fibrillation, energy levels between 75–200 J biphasic will be necessary. In a patient with an excessive thoracic diameter, 200–300 J biphasic may be ncessary

---

FIGURE 2.16 Guide for Succesful Cardioversion

Care should be taken to avoid exposure to high flow oxygen. In an oxygen risk environment, electrical sparking from the paddles could ignite a fire. Fortunately, there are no reports of fires occurring when using the adhesive pads.. If first shock is not successful, examine the pads for optimal location and adherence. If necessary, replace pads. Consider repositioning anterior pad to optimize the direction of current flow delivered. With proper technique and safety precautions, cardioversion remains an effective, safe, low risk, economical and well-tolerated procedure [4] (Fig. 2.16) [26] (Fig. 2.17).

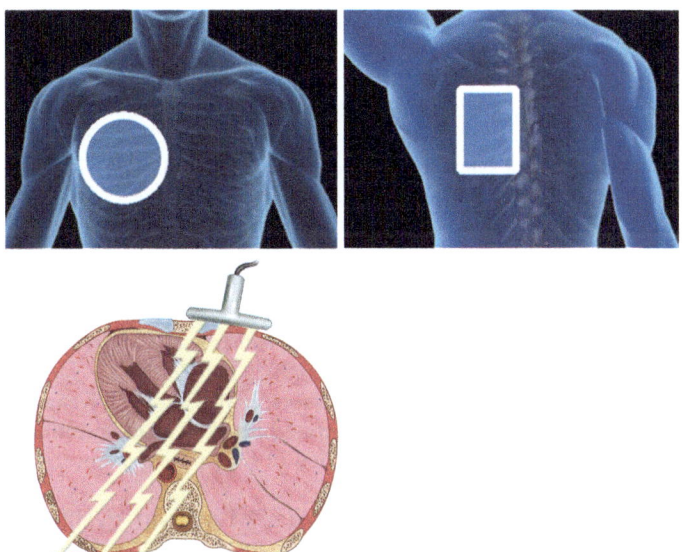

FIGURE 2.17 Optimal Energy Vector for Cardioversion

References

1. Abilgard C. Tentamina electica in animalibus institua. Societatis Medicae Havniensis Collectanea. 1775;2:157.
2. Bartoletti A, Alboni P, Ammirati F, Brignole M, Del Rosso A, Foglia Manzillo F, et al. The Italian Protocol: a simplified head-up tilt testing potentiated with oral nitroglycerin to assess patients with unexplained syncope. Europace. 2000;2(4): 339–42.
3. Benditt D, Blanc J, Brignole M, Sutton R. The evaluation of treatment of syncope. A handbook for clinical practice. Oxford: Wiley-Blackwell; 2006.

4. Botkina S, Dhanekulaa L, Olshansky B. Outpatient cardioversion of atrial arrhythmias: efficacy, safety, and costs. Am Heart J. 2003;145(2):233–8.

5. Brignole M, Alboni P, Benditt D, Bergfeldt L, Blanc J, Bloch Thomsen P, et al. Guidelines on management (diagnosis and treatment) of syncope. Eur Heart J. 2001;22(15):1256–306.

6. Farwell D, Freemantle N, Sulke N. The clinical impact of implantable loop recorders in patients with syncope. Eur Heart J. 2006;27:351–6.

7. Ganzeboom KS, Mairuhu G, Reitmas J, Linzer M, Weiling W, van Dijk N. Lifetime cumulative incidence of syncope int the general population: a study of 549 Dutch subjects aged 35–60 years. J Cardiovasc Electrophysiol. 2006;17(11):1172–6.

8. Gieroba Z, Newton J, Parry S, Norton M, Lawson J, Kenny R. Unprovoked and glyceryl trinitrate-provoked head-up tilt table test is safe in older people: a review of 10 years' experience. J Am Geriatr Soc. 2004;52(11):1913–5.

9. Glotzer T, Daoud E, Wyse D, Singer D, Ezekowitz M, Hilker C, et al. The relationship between daily atrial tachyarrhythmia burden from implantable device diagnostics and stroke risk: the TRENDS study. Circ Arrhythm Electrophysiol. 2009;2:474–80.

10. Kenny R, Ingram A, Bayliss J, Sutton R. Head-up tilt: a useful test for investigating unexplained syncope. Lancet. 1986;1: 1352–5.

11. Kenny R, O'Shea D, Parry S. The Newcastle Protocols for head-up tilt table testing in the diagnosis of vasovagal syncope, carotid sinus hypersensitivity and related disorders. Heart. 2000; 83:564–9.

12. Leitch J, Klein GJ, Yee R, Leather RA, Kim YH. Syncope associated with supraventricular tachycardia. An expression of tachycardia rate or vasomotor response? Circulation. 1992;85: 1064–71.

13. Lown B. Defibrillation and cardioversion. Cardiovasc Res. 2002; 55(2):220–4.

14. Lown B, Amarasingham R, Neuman J. New method for terminating cardiac arrhythmias. Use of synchronized capacitor discharge. JAMA. 1962;182:548–55.

15. McIntosh S, Kenny R. Carotid sinus syndrome in the elderly. J Royal Soc Med. 1994;87:798–800.

16. Moya A et al. Guidelines for the diagnosis and management of syncope (version 2009). European Heart Journal 2009;30: 2631–2671. doi:10.1093/eurheartj/ehp298.

17. Numeroso F, et al. Evaluation of the current prognostic role of heart diseases in the history of patients with syncope. Europace. 2014;16(9):1379–83. doi:10.1093/europace/eut402. Epub 2014 Jan 31.

18. Parry S, Reeve P, Lawson J, Shaw F, Davison J, Norton M, et al. The Newcastle protocols 2008: an update on head-up tilt table testing and the management of vasovagal syncope and related disorders. Heart. 2009;95(5):416–20.

19. Richardson D, Bexton R, Shaw F, Steen N, Bond J, Kenny R. Complications of carotid sinus massage – a prospective series of older patients. Age Ageing. 2000;29(5):413–7.

20. Roth N. First stammering of the heart: Ludwig's kymograph. Med Instrum. 1978;12:348.

21. Sanna T, et al. Cryptogenic Stroke and Underlying Atrial Fibrillation N Engl J Med 2014;370:2478–86.

22. Sun BC, Emond J. Direct medical costs of syncope – related hospitalizations in the United States. Am J Cardiol. 2005;95(5):668–71.

23. Tan M, Parry S. Vasovagal syncope in the older patient. J Am Coll Cardiol. 2008;51:599–606.

24. Timoteo AT, Oliveira MM, Feliciano J, Antunes E, Nogueira da Silva M, Silva S, et al. Head-up tilt testing with different nitroglycerin dosages: experience in elderly patients with unexplained syncope. Europace. 2008;10(9):1091–4.

25. Medtronic Carelink Event Monitor Sample Report. www.medtronicdiagnostics.com/wcm/groups/mdtcom_sg/@mdt/documents/documents/reveal-linq-system-followup.pdf. 2014. Retrieved from www.medtronic.com.

26. Zoll Medical Corporation. Technical note: keys to successful cardioversion. 2009. August 2013, from www.zoll.com/uploaded-files/public_site/core_technologies/cardioversion

Chapter 3
A Brief Overview of Supraventricular Tachycardias

Spencer Rosero

Supraventricular tachycardias are a group of arrhythmias that include atrio-ventricular nodal tachycardias (AVNRT), atrial tachycardia, and atrio-ventricular reentry tachycardias (AVRT) including Wolff-Parkinson-White Syndrome. The purpose of this chapter is to provide a basic overview of the mechanisms, management and practical considerations in the electrophysiology laboratory.

Atrioventricular Nodal Reentry

The most common type of SVT is atrioventricular nodal reentry (AVNRT), accounting for the majority of diagnosed SVT in patients under 50 years, with a higher prevalence in women compared to men. Quality of life has also been shown to be affected in various populations [1, 2]. Clinical ECG demonstrates a short RP, narrow complex tachycardia with evidence of retrograde conduction seen as a pseudo S wave with a superior axis P waves (Fig. 3.1).

S. Rosero, MD
Department of Cardiology, Hereditary Arrhythmia Clinic,
University of Rochester Medical Center, Rochester, NY, USA
e-mail: spencer_rosero@urmc.rochester.edu

D.T. Huang, T. Prinzi (eds.), *Clinical Cardiac*
Electrophysiology in Clinical Practice, In Clinical Practice,
DOI 10.1007/978-1-4471-5433-4_3,
© Springer-Verlag London 2015

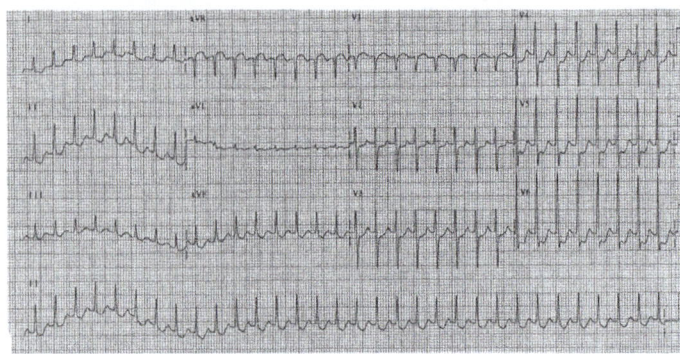

FIGURE 3.1   ECG of AVNRT. Notice retrograde P waves forming a pseudo S pattern in several leads

This short RP tachycardia involves a reentry mechanism within the AV node and is based on the concept of dual AV nodal physiology. The reentrant circuit is dependent on the presence of at least two functional pathways with differing refractoriness and conduction properties. Typical AVNRT, the most frequent form, uses the slow pathway for antegrade conduction, and the fast pathway for retrograde limb to complete the circuit and is classically triggered by an APC blocking in the fast pathway but conducting slowly down the slow pathway allowing retrograde recovery of the fast pathway to produce a closed loop (Fig. 3.2) [3, 4].

The two pathways do not seem separable by pathologic examination but the characteristics are encoded within the cellular distribution, and the characteristics for electrophysiology properties are functional [4–6]. The differentiation of function within the AV node was originally discovered from analyzing atrial pacing data using progressively shorter atrial extrastimuli cycle lengths (A1-A2) and measuring the A-H conduction times, during which it was noted that a large "jump" of at least 50 ms occurred at a specific 10 ms decrement in A1-A2 cycle length after which the resumption of gradual normal decremental conduction would continue on a different slope (Fig. 3.3). This reproducible finding confirmed

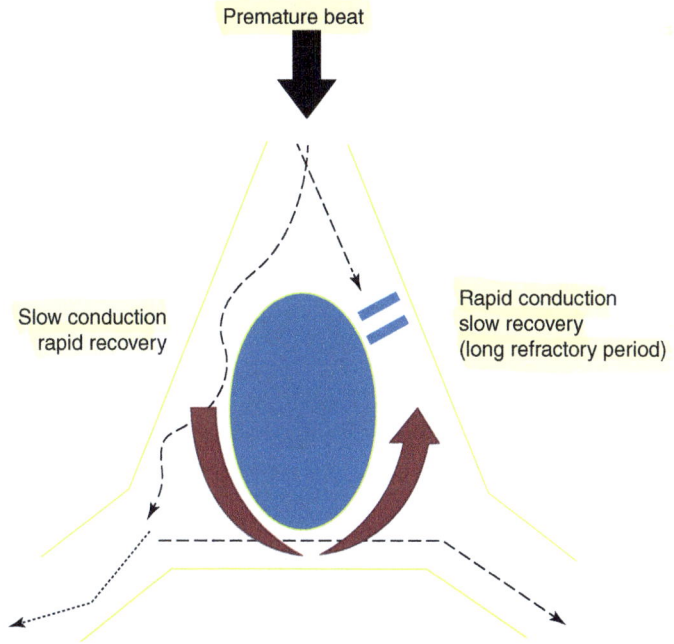

FIGURE 3.2 Diagram of dual pathway physiology within the AV node and initiation via an APC

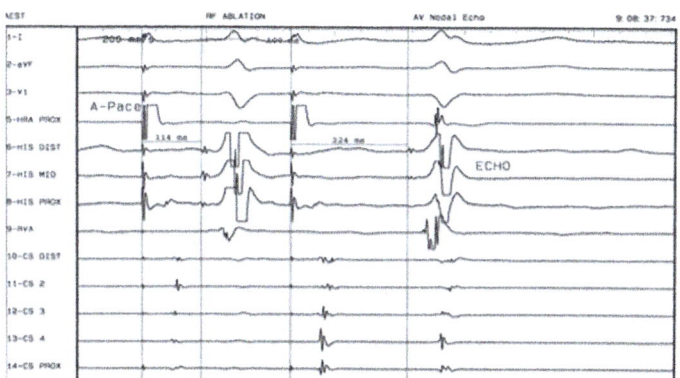

FIGURE 3.3 Paced atrial extrastimuli with subsequent "jump" in AH interval and one beat reentry. This is referred to as an echo

the functional presence of dual pathway physiology and provides the substrate for a reentry based tachycardia such as AVNRT. This mechanism also explains the surface ECG findings of an APC with sudden PR prolongation preceding initiation of a short RP tachycardia with evidence of retrograde P wave conduction. The intracardiac findings confirm a jump in AH interval meeting the dual pathway criteria with initiation of a short RP tachycardia.

The atrial electrogram on the His catheter is earliest since the return limb in the typical form involves the anterior pathway located close to the anteroseptal region.

The fast and slow pathways are considered to anatomically located within the triangle of Koch during which the earliest retrograde conduction to the atrium is noted. In typical AVNRT, the earliest retrograde atrial activation EGM is noted in the apex of the triangle, and in the OS of the coronary sinus during the atypical form. It is important to note that not all cases of AVNRT demonstrate clear dual AV nodal physiology during baseline EP studies, since the "jump" is heavily influenced by timing and autonomic tone.

Clinical Presentation

Patients with AVNRT often present with a history of paroxysmal palpitations, that may be triggered after bending down to pickup a heavy object, or preceded by a sensation of single "skipped beats". It is interesting to note that many adolescent patients instinctively perform their own vagal maneuvers to terminate the SVT including bearing down or less commonly, standing on their head terminating the tachycardia via vagal like mechanism. Adults may describe a history of palpitations during their teenage years, the frequency of which may have decreased for many years, only to return later in life. While the tachycardia cycle length may decrease in a subgroup of patients with age, the ability to tolerate the fast rates may not. Common symptoms include sudden onset and termination, sensation of racing or palpitations, chest heaviness or unusual sensation in neck and throat prompting a cough. While the

SVT may last only minutes, it may be prolonged and incessant prompting an emergency room visit. Intravenous adenosine is often used in the pre-hospital and hospital setting with excellent success in terminating the tachycardia.

Clinical Management

There are three decision pathways: Observation, Pharmacologic, and Catheter ablation. The individual patient's circumstances need to be included in the process. For example, a single episode of SVT and no history of symptoms may benefit from observation or event monitoring with no pharmacologic or invasive intervention. Catheter ablation is generally curative and is the preferred path for patients with recurrent episodes that are symptomatic, limited by possibility of having prolonged episodes requiring emergency services, and/or occupation that may increase patient risk for injury should he or she develop sustained SVT that is symptomatic. Pharmacologic management primarily rely on drugs such as beta receptor and calcium channel antagonists that modulate AV node function to reduce the probability of SVT events over long periods of time. The next level of pharmacologic intervention would include antiarrhythmics such as flecainide or propafenone, which concomitantly have a higher side effect profile.

Electrophysiology Study and Ablation

Several forms of AVNRT have been described during EP studies including slow-fast (typical) and fast-slow (atypical). The correct diagnosis is critical to determining if and where an RF ablation should be delivered. The goal is to eliminate the appropriate limb of the reentry circuit while minimizing risk to the normal conduction system. When performing the EP study for SVT, it is important to maintain a systematic approach to avoid missing key maneuvers and improving your diagnostic accuracy. We recommend that physicians customize and adopt a framework on which to approach all EP studies. The following is only an example of possible considerations during an EP study:

1. Document baseline sinus rhythm, AH, HV intervals. Any preexcitation?, is the AV conduction normal?
2. 1:1 A-V conduction
3. AV node function – Effective refractory periods using programmed stimulation
4. Any evidence of dual AV nodal physiology? (Fig. 3.3)
5. 1:1 V-A conduction: Is it concentric? Is it decremental?
6. Parahisian pacing (Fig. 3.4)
7. Attempt burst pacing and varying atrial and ventricular extrastimuli.
8. Add agents such as isoproterenol or atropine to alter autonomic tone to increase the probability of inducing SVT.

In typical AVNRT, the ECG reveals a short RP narrow complex regular tachycardia in which the P wave is buried within the terminal segment of the QRS complex and not clearly visible. Intracardiac electrograms demonstrate that the earliest retrograde activation is often seen on the His

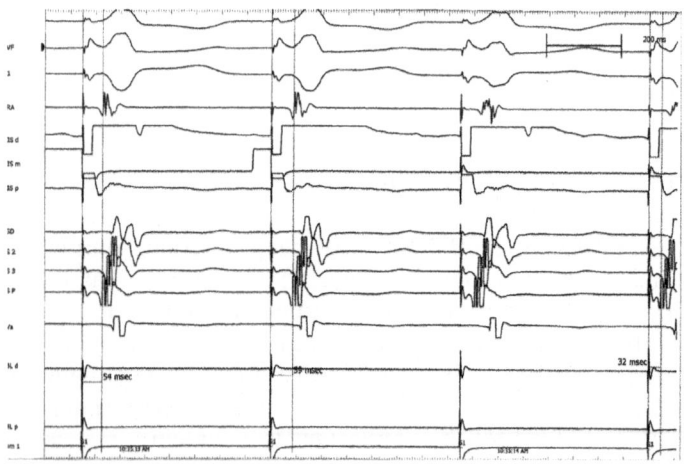

FIGURE 3.4 Example of ParaHisian pacing

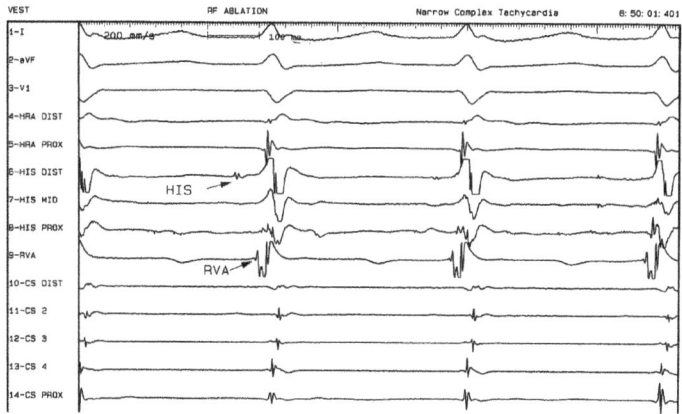

FIGURE 3.5 Atrioventricular nodal reentry tachycardia

Bundle electrode, though it may be occasionally seen earlier along the posterior septum (Fig. 3.5). The QA interval is relatively short. One must always consider the less probable presence of a left sided fast pathway.

Pacing maneuvers during tachycardia are powerful tools for correctly diagnosing the circuit. For example, rapid ventricular pacing causing dissociation between the atrium and ventricle provides a clue. In this setting, the atrial cycle length remains unchanged thus ruling out AVRT as the etiology of the ongoing tachycardia but does not rule out arrhythmias such as atrial tachycardia. Another maneuver during 1:1 conduction involves introducing single premature ventricular beats at a time during His refractoriness and determining if it resets the atrial activation. Parahisian pacing also aids in determining the presence of a concealed septal bypass tract [7, 8].

It is important to recognize that there is a small but real risk of damaging the AV node fast pathway causing high grade AV block that may be irreversible. Fluoroscopic views maximizing the distance between the anteroseptum and the posteroseptal region near the coronary sinus where the slow pathway is localized reduces risk. Additionally, 3D mapping in which the His bundle is carefully marked can reduce risk.

During RF delivery, monitoring VA conduction during junctional beats as well as the A-H-V conduction during sinus will provide clues to unintended conduction system damage.

Atrial Tachycardia

Atrial tachycardias originate from cells depolarizing within the atria and function independently of the AV node conduction system and ventricle. The anatomic site of origin can be anywhere in the left and right atria. An atrial tachycardia may originate from one or more foci and presents on ECG as an SVT with evidence of p waves that may or may not have a fixed relationship to the QRS. The surface ECG usually reveals p waves with vectors different from the sinus node activation pattern (Figs. 3.6 and 3.7). Normal sinus rhythm presents with P waves that are positive in I, II, and negative in AVR. A tachycardia originating near the sinus node or from within the sinus tissue, it would appear similar to sinus activation pattern and the possibility of sinus node reentry should be considered. The atrial cycle length of atrial tachycardias are generally longer than atrial flutter cycle lengths that are often ~200–250 ms. The P wave morphology of atrial tachycardias often appear similar to sinus P waves versus peaked saw tooth pattern waves seen in atrial flutter. On occasion, we find that what appeared to be an atrial tachycardia on surface ECG was found to be an atypical atrial flutter during an EP study.

The mechanism may consist of a focal automaticity, intra-atrial reentry, or triggered automaticity. While Focal automaticity is generally resistant to termination by burst pacing, reentry or triggered automaticity based tachycardias are often induced and terminated by burst pacing.

Atrial tachycardias may occur in children for a variety of reasons including congenital heart disease, particularly

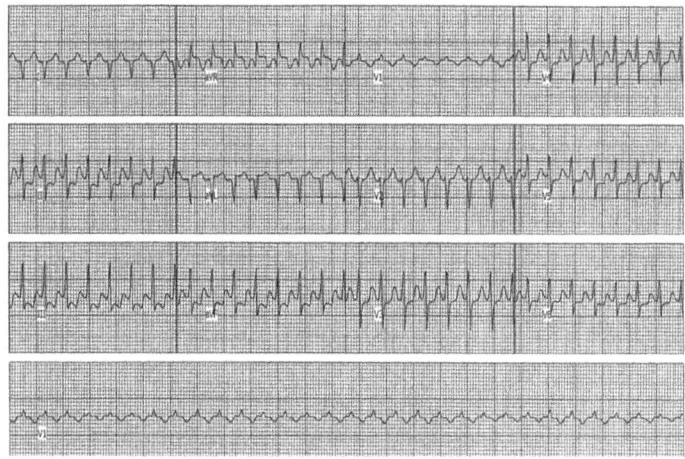

FIGURE 3.6 Standard 12 lead ECG example of atrial tachycardia

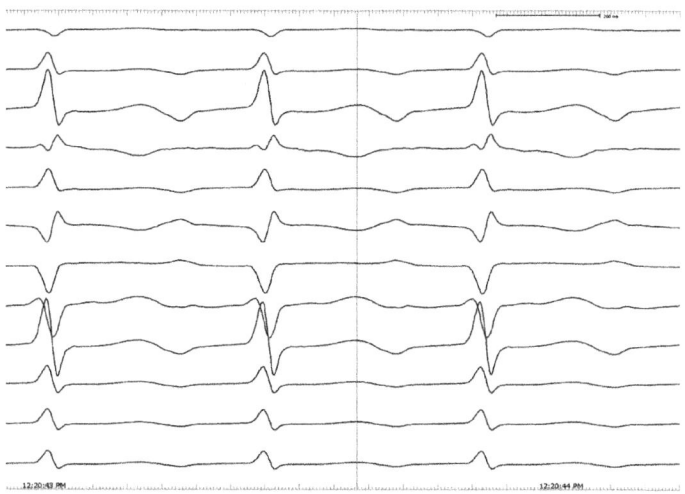

FIGURE 3.7 Magnified 12 Lead to discern P wave activity

in the very young with decreasing prevalence with age. It may be seen in adults over time as a lone problem or accompanying myocarditis, thyroid disease, both acute and chronic pulmonary disease, and in patient with cardiomyopathies.

Clinical Presentation

Patient often present with a chief complaint of palpitations or 'skipping'. Their ECG may reveal rates that may be within the range of normal sinus rhythm or sinus tachycardia up to rates around 180 bpm. The intermediate rates may make it hard to discern between sinus or atrial tachycardia, though one would expect that the setting in which the ECG is obtained will improve the specificity. For example, sitting quietly in the office with sudden onset of tachycardia at 165 bpm 1:1 AV conduction would be more consistent with an atrial tachycardia than sinus tachycardia. However, these tachycardias present as persistent and stable rhythms at rates mimicking sinus tachycardia and difficult to discern without a 12 lead ECG. The differential diagnosis of underlying etiology requires a detailed patient history that may suggest an acute disease process such as pulmonary embolus, RV failure, thyroid disease, pulmonary disease.

Clinical Management

The treatment of underlying cause is naturally a first step for those patients in which direct trigger is found. However, the vast majority of patients will need to be treated with a tiered pharmacologic approach that may start with beta blockade or antiarrhythmic to control the frequency, duration, and symptoms associated with an atrial tachycardia while minimizing side effects from the drugs themselves. If there is a focal atrial morphology, then radiofrequency ablation of the site is a preferred strategy with a high probability of cure.

Electrophysiology Study and Ablation

Review of the 12 lead ECG often provides information regarding location and cycle length of the tachycardia. The consideration of location should be done prior to starting the procedure to avoid surprises and determine equipment that may be needed. The main consideration is whether the tachycardia is located in the left atrium or pulmonary veins which would require transeptal approach and anticoagulation. 3-D electro-anatomical and non-contact mapping is critical to localizing the circuit or focus while minimizing radiation exposure from fluoroscopy. There are several 3D mapping systems available which continuously improve their technology making mapping more efficient and accurate [9–11]. The approach to the EP study for atrial tachycardias assumes that single and 12 lead ECGs (Fig. 3.3) have been thoroughly reviewed with a differential diagnosis in place to help guide the strategy. During the EP study, one should consider the following:

1. Document baseline sinus rhythm, AH, HV intervals. Any preexcitation?, is the AV conduction normal?
2. Select best leads to view P wave morphology on the EP recording system (Figs. 3.6 and 3.7)
3. If in AT where does the 12 lead ECG localize the origin to?
4. 1:1 A-V conduction during tachycardia – Consider adenosine, and review baseline variable conduction or use ventricular burst pacing to separate A-V relationship ruling out AVRT (Figs. 3.8 and 3.9)
5. Attempt to determine mechanism : focal, triggered automaticity, or reentry. Use pacing maneuvers to attempt entrainment with concealed fusion to determine if a reentry mechanism is noted.
6. Characterize AV node function – Effective refractory periods using programmed stimulation should be done as part of any EP study
7. Any evidence of dual AV nodal physiology or accessory pathways?

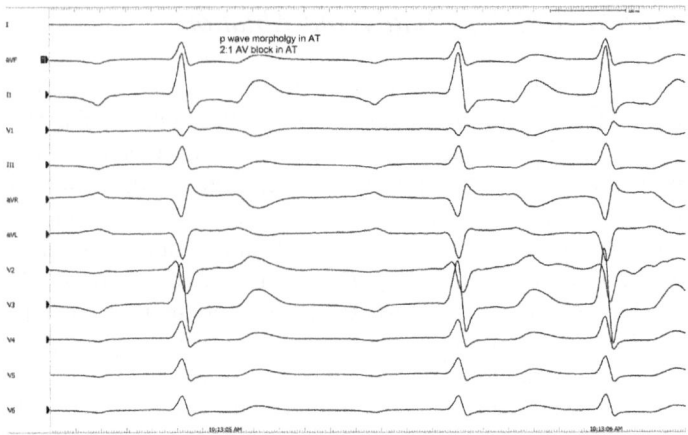

FIGURE 3.8 2:1 block during atrial tachycardia confirm A-V dissociation ruling out AVRT

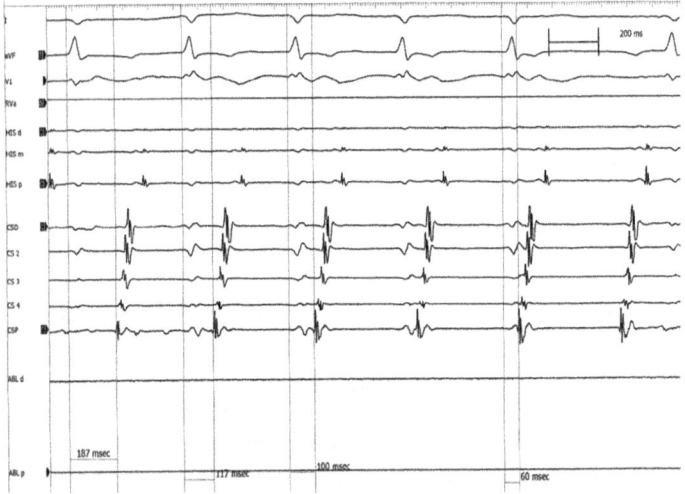

FIGURE 3.9 Intracardiac recording confirming 12 lead of A-V dissociation during tachycardia. Note that the earliest atrial signal is located in the proximal coronary sinus electrode. This only narrows down location based on current electrodes. One can only say that the earliest atrial activation from the electrodes current in place is the proximal CS

8. 1:1 V-A conduction: Is it concentric? Is it decremental?
9. Add agents such as isoproterenol or atropine to alter autonomic tone to increase the probability of inducing SVT.
10. Where is earliest atrial signal compared to surface P wave?
11. Consider phrenic nerve injury and confirm with pacing before ablating [12]

A patient may have an atrial tachycardia but may also develop other lab induced tachycardias including AVNRT, atrial fibrillation, or atrial flutter that may or may not have clinical significance.

The mapping of focal atrial tachycardias integrates electrogram analysis, timing, and is best done by utilizing 3D electro-anatomical mapping systems to store geospatial points and minimize fluoroscopy. In focal atrial tachycardias, we often use a triggered mode screen format which provides a visual trigger on each atrial beat and allows us to map quickly obtaining the earliest atrial signal on the distal electrode of the ablation catheter compared to the surface P wave. Choosing the right reference on 3D mapping is important. It is important to always consider that an early atrial endocardial signal in single chamber mapping, for example the right atrium, may be earliest on a 3D map of the right atrium but later than the surface P wave if the origin is in the left atrium, right superior pulmonary vein. The reference electrode chosen determines accuracy of origin as well as diagnosis when it comes to optimizing 3D mapping. There are various 3D mapping systems available. Figures 3.10 and 3.11 demonstrate EGM mapping of an atrial tachycardia localized to a site posterior to the coronary sinus os.

SVT Mapping Considerations

Different 3D mapping strategies will be utilized depending on the diagnosis of the SVT.

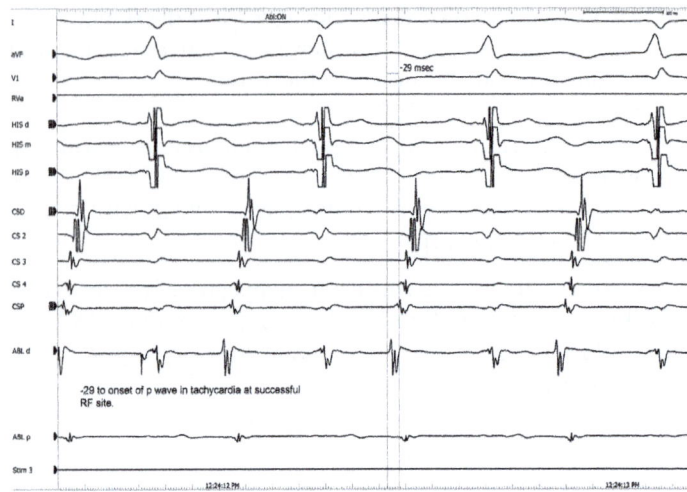

FIGURE 3.10 EGM mapping of atrial tachycardia. Successful termination of the tachycardia was achieved using the earliest atrial signal is seen at the distal electrode of the ablation catheter (ABL d) at a location posterior to the coronary sinus and 29 ms earlier than the onset of the surface P wave. It is directly under the Tricuspid valve – far field R waves can be seen

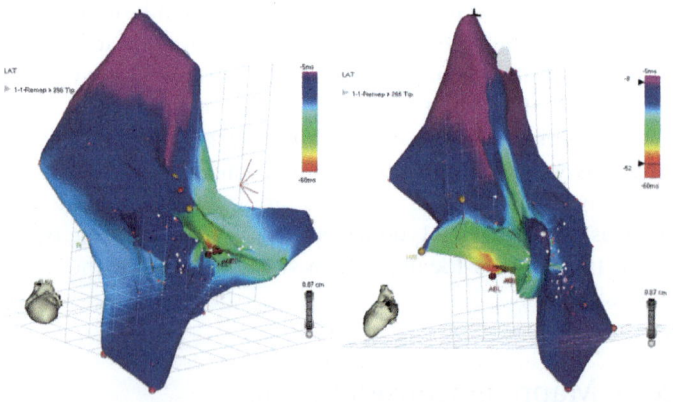

FIGURE 3.11 LAO and PA views of Carto 3D Map of the right atrium and earliest EGM. The site of ablation is denoted by dark red points marked Abl

AVNRT

In most cases, AVNRT 3D mapping will be only anatomical. Some operators may prefer to collect an entire right atrial anatomical geometry, marking out the tricuspid valve in detail. Others may choose to simply mark important anatomical sites with location tags and not collect the actual chamber. In either case, the most important anatomical marker in AVNRT mapping is a detailed His bundle, to prevent AV block. Marking the CS ostium is also helpful for safety. If multiple ablations are required to eliminate the slow pathway, it is helpful to use a different color tag to mark the site of effective ablation and places where multiple junctional beats were observed. In the event of a recovery of the slow pathway during the post-ablation testing phase, the electrophysiologist will be able to easy navigate back to the spot in question. Due to the sensitivity of the structures in the triangle of Koch, it is also recommended to use respiratory gating technology on the 3D map, and to take all anatomical tags consistently at end expiration. (Respirations can account for up to 5 mm of inaccuracy in 3D maps, and 5 mm can make a critical difference when trying to avoid AV block.)

AVRT

Mapping a pathway can be done in multiple ways. In its simplest form, the 3D mapper can simply use location tags to mark areas of interest (AV fusion, AP potentials), so that the EP can return to those locations after exploring the entire valve. Electroanatomic (EA) mapping can also be beneficial. Window of interest choices must be made in order to properly map. It is usually best to map accessory pathways while pacing. If the pathway conducts both antegradely and retrogradely, pacing from either chamber will work; if the pathway only conducts retrogradely, you must pace from the ventricle. It is usually best to use the pacing spike of the catheter you are pacing as the "time zero" reference, and then map to the distal chamber (e.g., use RV catheter for reference while RV pacing, and annotate on atrial electrograms). When mapping this way, note that all times will be positive (no negative window). Therefore, a window of interest will usually be set at +20 to +150. See Chap. 4 on WPW for more on mapping AVRT.

Atrial Tachycardia

Atrial tachycardias can be surprisingly difficult to map. Challenges include previous ablations (AT is often present post AF ablation; see AF chapter for more on post-AF LA AT), areas of scar, multiple tachycardias (or multifocal AT), varying cycle lengths, and difficulty inducing and sustaining AT. Sometimes differentiating mechanism (automatic, trigger, microreentry, or macroreentry) can be problematic. Mapping reentrant atrial tachycardias is covered in the atrial flutter chapter. But because triggered activity and microreentry can mask as macroreentry, and we recommend approaching the mapping for AT in the same way as mapping a macroreentrant tachycardia. By using the DePonti algorithm for calculating the window of interest, focal, microreentrant, and macroreentrant possibilities will all be taking into account during the EA mapping. If reentry has been entirely ruled out by pacing maneuvers, the window can simply be set to have the backwards interval timed at 80–100 ms before p wave onset. If p waves cannot be observed, it is best to administer adenosine. The window of interest's relationship to the p wave is critical to accurately mapping the AT.

It is important to recognize that no matter how high density and rapid the mapping system may be, 3D mapping will be impossible with multifocal AT and extremely difficult with rapidly changing ATs.

References

1. Suenari KJ, et al. Gender differences in the clinical characteristics and atrioventricular nodal conduction properties in patients with atrioventricular nodal reentrant tachycardia. J Cardiovasc Electrophysiol. 2010;21(10):1114–9.
2. Walfridsson U, et al. Wolff-Parkinson-White syndrome and atrioventricular nodal re-entry tachycardia in a Swedish population: consequences on health-related quality of life. Pacing Clin Electrophysiol. 2009;32(10):1299–306.
3. Jackman WM, et al. Treatment of supraventricular tachycardia due to atrioventricular nodal reentry, by radiofrequency catheter ablation of slow-pathway conduction. N Engl J Med. 1992;327(5):313–8.
4. Stabile G, et al. The predictive value of junctional beats during the radiofrequency transcatheter ablation of the slow pathway of the nodal reentry circuit. G Ital Cardiol. 1999;29(5):549–54.
5. Demosthenes GK, et al. Atrioventricular nodal reentrant tachycardia. Circulation. 2010;122:831–40.
6. Demosthenes GK, et al. Classification of electrophysiological types of atrioventricular nodal re-entrant tachycardia: a reappraisal. Europace. 2013;15:1231–40.
7. Reddy V, et al. Para-Hisian entrainment: a novel pacing maneuver to differentiate orthodromic atrioventricular reentrant tachycardia from atrioventricular nodal reentrant tachycardia. J Cardiovasc Electrophysiol. 2003;14(12):1321–8.
8. Hiaro K, et al. Para-Hisian pacing. Circulation. 1996;94(5):1027–35.
9. Wu RC, Berger R, Calkins H. Catheter ablation of atrial flutter and macroreentrant atrial tachycardia. Curr Opin Cardiol. 2002;17(1):58–64.
10. Chen SA, Chiang CE, Yang CJ, et al. Sustained atrial tachycardia in adult patients. Electrophysiological characteristics, pharmacological response, possible mechanisms, and effects of radiofrequency ablation. Circulation. 1994;90(3):1262–78.
11. Marcus W, et al. Catheter ablation of non-sustained focal right atrial tachycardia guided by virtual non-contact electrograms. Europace. 2011;13:876–82.
12. Huemer M, Wutzler A, Parwani AS, et al. Mapping of the left-sided phrenic nerve course in patients undergoing left atrial catheter ablations. Pacing Clin Electrophysiol. PACE:2014.

Chapter 4
Wolff-Parkinson-White (WPW) Syndrome

Jeffrey M. Vinocur

WPW, in its full form, is the combination of ventricular pre-excitation on ECG plus palpitations (due to orthodromic AVRT). Often the term "Asymptomatic WPW" is used, somewhat confusingly, to refer to the finding of a WPW-type baseline ECG without any subjective or documented arrhythmia. In either case, the anatomic abnormality is that of an accessory AV pathway with antegrade (and almost always retrograde) conduction.

These pathways can support several arrhythmias (orthodromic AVRT, antidromic AVRT, and pathway-to-pathway reentry in patients with multiple pathways), and act as bystanders to others (most often atrial arrhythmias, although AVNRT with bystander pathway conduction can occur). SVT in the form of orthodromic AVRT is by far the most common manifestation. However, special attention must be drawn to the entity of atrial fibrillation with "bystander" conduction down the accessory pathway, because this can lead to sudden death, even in previously asymptomatic persons. Finally, there is one non-arrhythmic manifestation of WPW, that of left

J.M. Vinocur, MD
Pediatric Cardiology, Golisano Children's Hospital,
University of Rochester, Rochester, NY, USA
e-mail: jeffrey_vinocur@urmc.rochester.edu

D.T. Huang, T. Prinzi (eds.), *Clinical Cardiac*   55
Electrophysiology in Clinical Practice, In Clinical Practice,
DOI 10.1007/978-1-4471-5433-4_4,
© Springer-Verlag London 2015

ventricular systolic dysfunction i.e. dyssynchrony-induced cardiomyopathy, similar to that induced by chronic right ventricular pacing.

Orthodromic AVRT is comparable between WPW and concealed accessory pathways, as described elsewhere. Antidromic AVRT is an uncommon wide-complex tachycardia using the accessory pathway antegrade and the AV node retrograde (see Fig. 4.1e). It is one of several so-called "pre-excited tachycardias," a category that also includes preexcited atrial fibrillation (see Fig. 4.1d) and almost every other form of SVT with bystander accessory pathway conduction (this can occur with AVNRT, atrial tachycardia, etc.).

The diagnosis of WPW is generally straightforward from the baseline ECG. Occasionally fusion between sinus and ventricular beats falsely gives the appearance of preexcitation (for example, late-coupled ventricular bigeminy can look

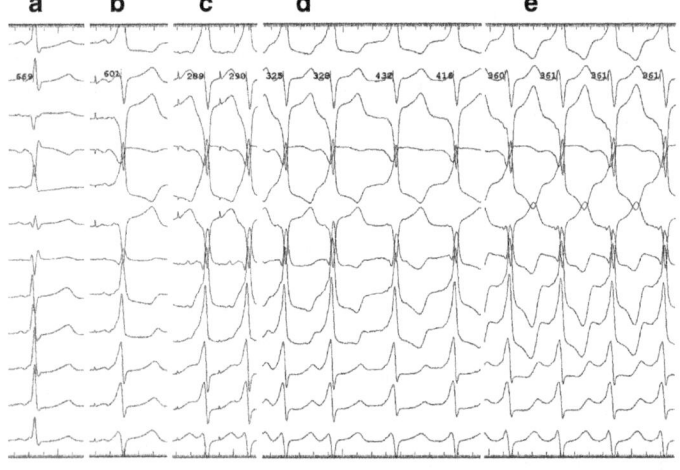

Figure 4.1 Surface ECG morphologies from a patient with WPW in different situations. (a) Sinus rhythm with subtle preexcitation, (b) Preexcitation maximized by slow atrial pacing plus adenosine, (c) Preexcitation maximized by rapid atrial pacing, (d) Irregular rhythm with variable degrees of preexcitation due to atrial fibrillation, (e) Regular rhythm with maximal preexcitation due to antidromic AVRT

like preexcitation alternans). Preexcitation can sometime be subtle (see Figs. 4.1a and 4.2), due to variable degrees of fusion between antegrade nodal and antegrade pathway conduction. Subtle preexcitation is more likely when the atrial depolarization reaches the pathway late (i.e. left-sided pathways), when nodal conduction is relatively rapid (i.e. young patient, elevated sympathetic tone), or when pathway conduction velocity is slow (particularly certain types of atypical pathways, discussed elsewhere). Antegrade pathway conduction can be absent or intermittent above certain atrial rates, depending on the effective refractory period of the pathway. Antegrade pathway conduction can also be absent

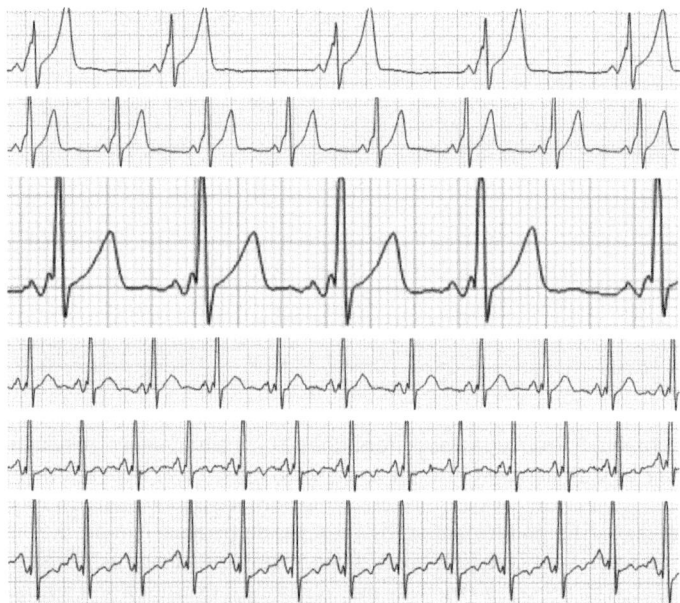

FIGURE 4.2 Series of strips from a single patient at various sinus rates, demonstrating variable degrees of fusion (related to autonomic effects on AV node conduction time, with antegrade pathway conduction present throughout); it is incorrect to use this type of "loss of preexcitation at faster heart rates" as a sign of a low-risk pathway

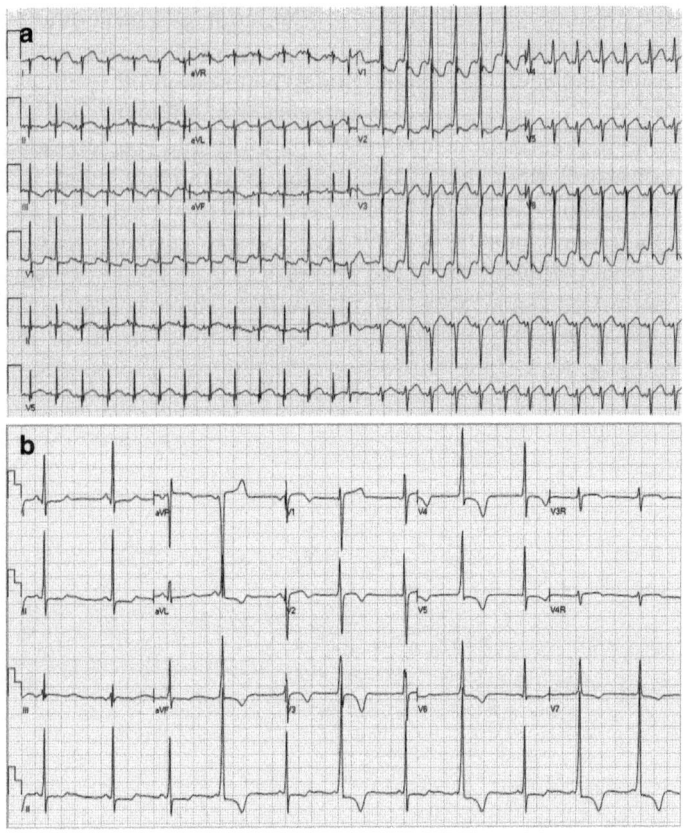

FIGURE 4.3 (a) Apparent "intermittent" preexcitation in a child with WPW, with narrow QRS due to repetitive concealed penetration of the His-Purkinje wavefront retrograde into the pathway, until a PAC disturbs the pattern and allows antegrade pathway conduction at the same sinus rate; this patient had "high-risk features" demonstrated at EP study. (b) Truly intermittent preexcitation (on a beat-by-beat basis) in a different patient with WPW and hypertrophic cardiomyopathy; note half-scale voltage for precordial leads

for reasons unrelated to pathway refractoriness (so-called "latent" pathways), including the phenomenon of concealed penetration of the His-Purkinje wavefront retrograde into the pathway (see Fig. 4.3a).

Additional rhythm recording (Holter, event recorder) may be indicated depending on symptoms. Echocardiography is indicated at baseline (to evaluate for comorbid structural heart disease, including Ebstein anomaly of the tricuspid valve, other forms of congenital heart disease, and hypertrophic cardiomyopathy) and perhaps periodically thereafter (to evaluate for ventricular dysfunction as mentioned above). Family screening is not generally recommended, as the recurrence risk in relatives is only modestly elevated (although certainly families with multiple affected members do occur).

Finally, the possibility of risk for sudden death must be considered. The mechanism of sudden death is believed to be that of rapidly conducted atrial fibrillation resulting in rapid irregular ventricular stimulation and eventually ventricular fibrillation. Patients with WPW are at increased risk for atrial fibrillation, even in the absence of structural heart disease. Therefore the risk of sudden death depends primarily on the antegrade conduction characteristics of the pathway. Patients with syncope, documented preexcited atrial fibrillation, multiple preexcited morphologies (since multiple pathways may alternate to allow rapid ventricular stimulation), and SVT (especially antidromic SVT) are at increased risk. Generally, older patients are believed to be at decreased risk, presumably because of survivor bias (i.e. those with rapid antegrade conduction would have presented with syncope or sudden death already).

A consensus statement from PACES (the Pediatric and Congenital EP Society) and HRS (the Heart Rhythm Society) provides guidance for the management of asymptomatic WPW in children and young adults [1]. Although studies differ about the exact magnitude of the risk for sudden death (e.g. between 0.1 and 5 per 1,000 patient-years), the guideline authors provide class IIa recommendations for risk stratification (acknowledging that no patient is at zero risk). The first step is non-invasive risk stratification, including ECG and if necessary exercise stress test, with the goal of identifying "abrupt and complete" loss of preexcitation at faster heart rates (felt to predict long accessory pathway refractory period). It is important to include only abrupt loss (i.e., in a single beat, see Figs. 4.3b and 4.4), and not be misled by

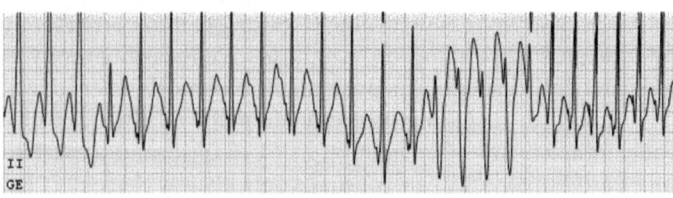

FIGURE 4.4 Strip from a patient with WPW undergoing exercise stress test. Preexcitation was present for the majority of the test, up through the first 3 beats on this strip. Then there is abrupt loss of preexcitation (in a single beat, associated with clear increase in PR) in the setting of sinus tachycardia to just over 200 bpm. After 11 beats of sinus tachycardia with antegrade nodal conduction, SVT begins, at a rate of nearly 300 bpm, with rate-related aberrancy for the first 4 beats

gradual fusion or day-to-day variation due to concealed retrograde penetration (see Figs. 4.2 and 4.3a). Only 10–20 % of patients will have convincingly reassuring non-invasive evaluations; invasive testing is recommended for the remainder. Invasive testing consists of diagnostic EP pacing study via either trans-esophageal or trans-venous route, with the goal being to induce sustained atrial fibrillation and measure the SPERRI (Shortest Pre-Excited R-R Interval, see Fig. 4.5). Assessment of SPERRI during atrial fibrillation is a stronger predictor than other pathway characteristics (such as SPERRI during rapid atrial pacing, or accessory pathway ERP, see Fig. 4.6) and should always be sought. Atrial fibrillation can be induced, with concerted effort, in well over 90 % of patients with WPW; prolonged rapid pacing just above atrial refractoriness usually suffices, but ramp pacing protocols and administration of adenosine can be helpful in difficult cases. SPERRI<250 ms, and especially <220 ms, is a predictor of higher risk for sudden death, and therefore an indication for prophylactic ablation (class IIa). The full algorithm (see Fig. 4.7) and accompanying text [1] capture additional nuance about balancing risks and benefits of ablation vs conservative management in various clinical situations.

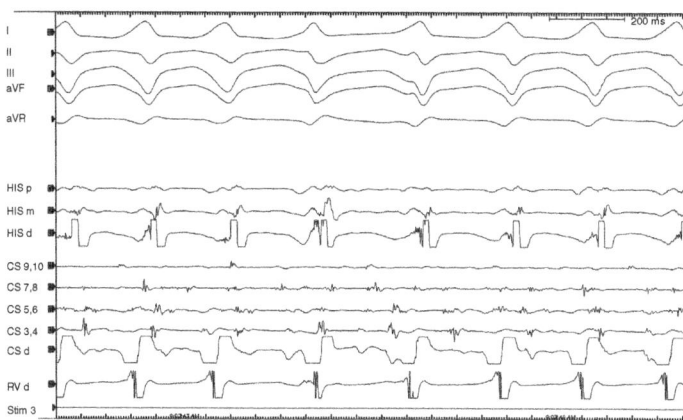

FIGURE 4.5 Atrial fibrillation with rapid antegrade pathway conduction; the shortest preexcited RR interval was 212 ms, suggestive of elevated risk for sudden death

Pharmacologic Management

For patients with WPW, medication is generally reserved for management of SVT (orthodromic AVRT) (Fig. 4.8) in patients felt not to be at risk for sudden death or who decline ablation. Because of some evidence that susceptibility to AVRT is itself a predictor of elevated risk (perhaps because rapid atrial stimulation during SVT can promote atrial fibrillation), ablation is used fairly liberally for patients with WPW and SVT. It is unknown if the risk stratification criteria for asymptomatic patients (see Fig. 4.7) can be extrapolated to patients symptomatic with palpitations or SVT.

For management of AVRT, unlike in patients with concealed accessory pathways (see elsewhere), digoxin and calcium-channel blockers are considered contraindicated in patients with WPW because of an association with sudden death (AV node blockade is felt to promote antegrade conduction down the pathway). Although the same concern theoretically exists for beta-blockers, these medications have

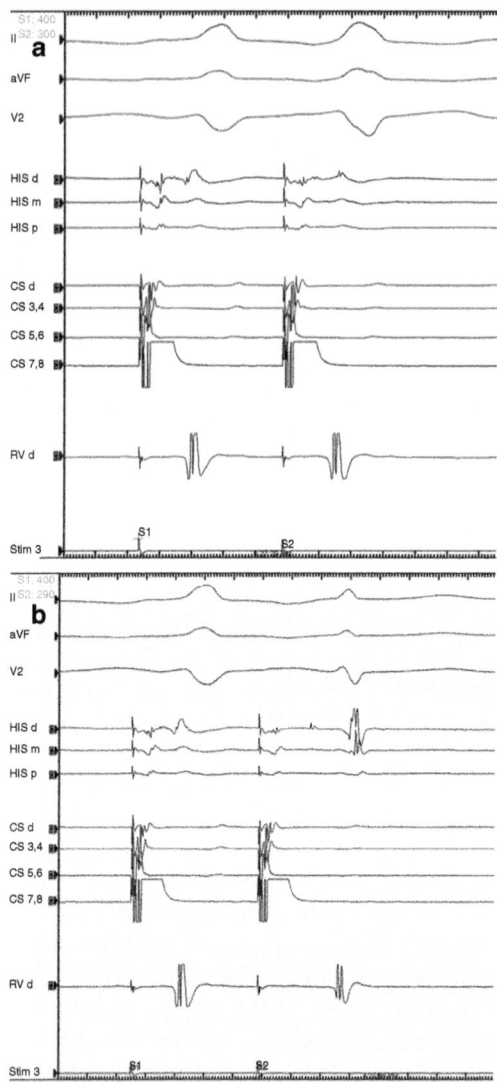

FIGURE 4.6 Surface and intracardiac electrograms from atrial extra-stimuli testing showing the accessory pathway effective refractory period with drive train S1 cycle length 400 ms and (**a**) S2 = 300 ms resulting in simultaneous antegrade pathway and nodal conduction with H-V interval < 0, compared to (**b**) S2 = 290 ms resulting in exclusively nodal conduction, with a much longer PR interval, normal H-V interval, and narrow QRS

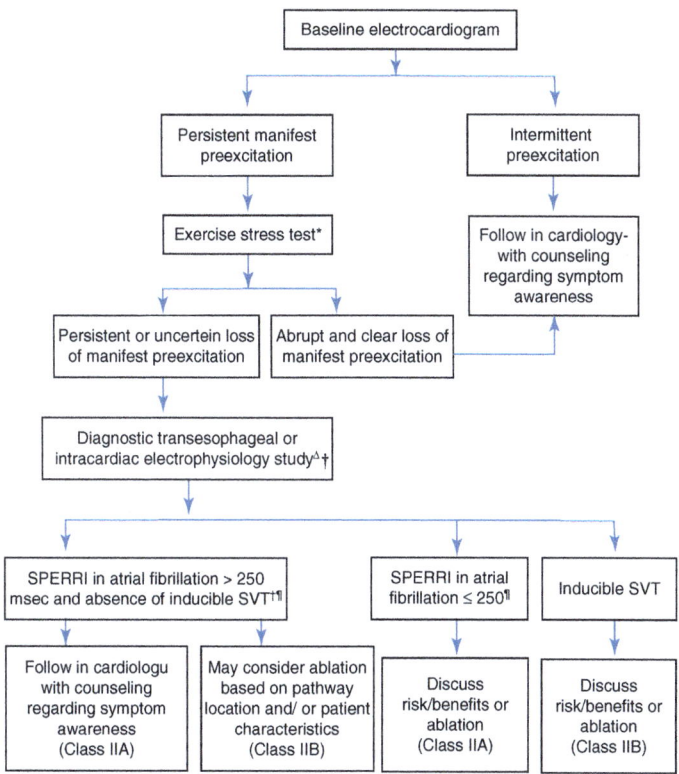

* Patients unable to perform an exercise stress test should undergo risk-stratification with an EP study

Δ Prior to invasive testing, patients and the parents/guardians should be counseled to discuss the risks and benefits of proceeding with invasive studies, risks of observation only, and risks of medication strategy.

† Patients participating at moderate-high level competitive sports should be counseled with regards to risk-benefit of ablation (Class IIA) and follow the 36th Bethesda Conference Guidelines[6]

¶ In the absence of inducible atrial fibrillation, the shortest pre-excited RR interval determined by rapid atrial pacing is a reasonable surrogate

FIGURE 4.7 Flowchart from PACES/HRS guidelines[1] for risk stratification of asymptomatic children and young adults with WPW (Reprinted with permission)

been used extensively in patients with WPW without convincing evidence for untoward effects. However, it is important to realize that beta-blockade does not reliably protect against rapidly conducted atrial fibrillation and sudden death in predisposed patients. Therefore beta-blockers are primarily

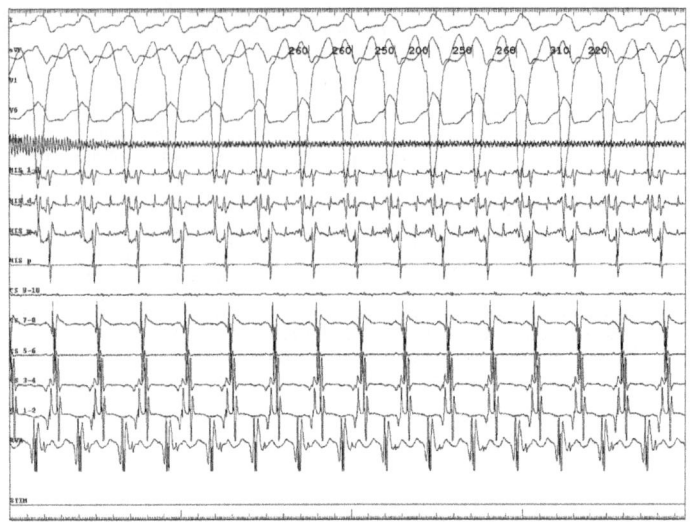

FIGURE 4.8 Orthodromic AVRT with LBBB aberrancy and earliest atrial activation at the His position, in a patient with an anteroseptal pathway

appropriate for management of SVT in patients felt to be at low risk for malignant arrhythmia.

Anti-arrhythmic agents with direct pathway activity (class I and class III agents) are also effective for treatment of AVRT, and are frequently used when beta-blockers are unsuccessful (or undesirable because of concern about malignant arrhythmia). Although catheter ablation is first-line for patients at high risk of malignant arrhythmia, class I and perhaps class III agents can be considered as alternatives (when ablation is refused or relatively contraindicated due to high-risk pathway location or extreme youth).

With regard to acute management, the same principles apply. For patients in AVRT, certainly intravenous calcium-channel blockers should be avoided. Adenosine and intravenous beta-blockers are reasonable, although appropriate resuscitation equipment should be available with adenosine because of its tendency to induce atrial fibrillation that could be rapidly conducted. Channel-active intravenous anti-arrhythmics can also be used, depending on local availability. When patients present in preexcited atrial fibrillation, emergent intervention is required, even if the rhythm is hemodynamically well tolerated. Immediate sedated cardioversion is prudent. Any delay (while awaiting NPO status, pharmacologic cardioversion, or EP lab activation) can be considered only in a closely-monitored setting with full resuscitation equipment immediately available.

Catheter-Based Management

Mapping

There are numerous approaches to mapping WPW, which offers flexibility to change strategies if one approach is not working well, but also can be confusing. It is important to understand no one approach will always be optimal; the choice should be individualized based on several factors.

All of the standard approaches for typical accessory pathways involve activation mapping around the tricuspid or mitral annulus, ideally with 3D mapping (which has been shown in some studies to improve success rates, and can minimize or even eliminate radiation exposure from fluoroscopy). Mapping can target the earliest atrial activation in any rhythm using the pathway retrograde (orthodromic AVRT, ventricular pacing) or earliest ventricular activation in any rhythm using the pathway antegrade (sinus, atrial pacing, antidromic AVRT). Each approach has its strengths and weaknesses, particularly because generally mapping and ablation should be performed in the same rhythm, leading to tradeoffs between facilitating mapping and facilitating safe and effective ablation (see Table 4.1).

One of the biggest pitfalls with mapping in WPW is the possibility of fusion between pathway and nodal conduction, which can occur when mapping in sinus, atrial paced, and ventricular paced rhythms. This can be partially avoided by carefully adjusting the rhythm to promote pathway conduction, for example by accelerating the pacing rate, changing the pacing

TABLE 4.1 Overview of the relative advantages of the various mapping approaches in WPW

Mapping target	Earliest A	Earliest A	Earliest V	Earliest V	Earliest V
Rhythm	Orthodromic-AVRT	V pacing	Sinus	A pacing	Antidromic-AVRT
Unambiguous map (no pathway/node fusion)	+++	+/++	+	+/++	+++
Crisp V electrograms (His-Purkinje activation)	++	+	+	+	+
Ability to assess node during ablation	+++	+	+/+++	+/+++	+
Stable catheter position during ablation	+/++	++	+++	++	+

In some situations, difficulties can be reduced by the techniques described in the text, indicated by +/++ or +/+++ in the table site to be closer to the pathway (best demonstrated by comparing the degree of preexcitation in right vs left atrial pacing at the same cycle length), or even administering medication (e.g. calcium-channel blocker). Mapping in AVRT completely eliminates this concern. Mapping in orthodromic AVRT provides another (smaller) advantage, which is that ventricular electrograms can be crisper (because of His-Purkinje activation) sometimes resulting in more easily interpreted signals. Of course, this assumes that AVRT can be readily induced and sustained; isoproterenol is often helpful in this regard. (Sometimes isoproterenol can be used briefly for induction of AVRT, and then discontinued to reduce cardiac motion while still allowing tachycardia to sustain.) The tradeoffs with different approaches are discussed further in section "Ablation".

Regardless of mapping strategy, it is critical to target the absolute earliest electrogram in the targeted chamber relative to a fixed reference point such as a coronary sinus bipole (for retrograde mapping) or a surface lead with a clearly identifiable deflection (for antegrade mapping). Although tempting, it can be quite misleading to target sites with short local A-V interval (for antegrade mapping) or V-A interval (for retrograde mapping); while this local "fusion" is frequently present at successful sites (see Figs. 4.9, 4.10c, 4.11b, 4.12b, 4.13a, 4.14, and 4.15a), it can also be present at distant sites where both components of the local electrogram are delayed by similar amounts.

Because almost all pathways are direct connections across the mitral or tricuspid annulus, interpretation of the maps is usually straightforward, with the earliest area being a point (or a small line running perpendicular to the atrioventricular groove), and with progressively later points on either side along the annulus (see Figs. 4.10a, 4.11a, and 4.12a). A broad early area suggests (1) imprecise electrogram interpretation that may benefit from careful manual review or switch to a different strategy, (2) fusion between pathway and nodal conduction, if plausible in the rhythm being used, (3) rarely, fusion between multiple pathways, or (4) that the true earliest area has not been explored, for example on the opposite side of the atrial septum, or (rarely) within an atrial appendage or coronary sinus.

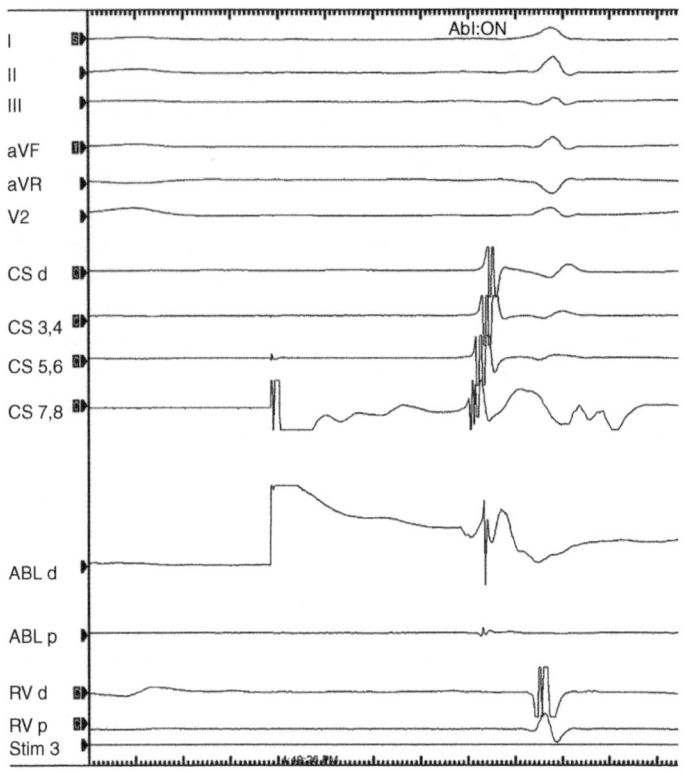

FIGURE 4.9 Surface and intracardiac electograms at the site of successful ablation from mapping earliest ventricular activation in sinus rhythm, note the very early ventricular component recorded from the ablation catheter. Artifact in CS7,8 and ABLd channels relates to onset of RF delivery

Entrainment

Although WPW supports SVT via a reentrant mechanism, it can be mapped like a focal tachycardia by following the activation pattern towards the earliest site (which should correspond to where the pathway crosses the atrioventricular groove). Thus, entrainment maneuvers are not critical to mapping of WPW. However, they can occasionally be useful

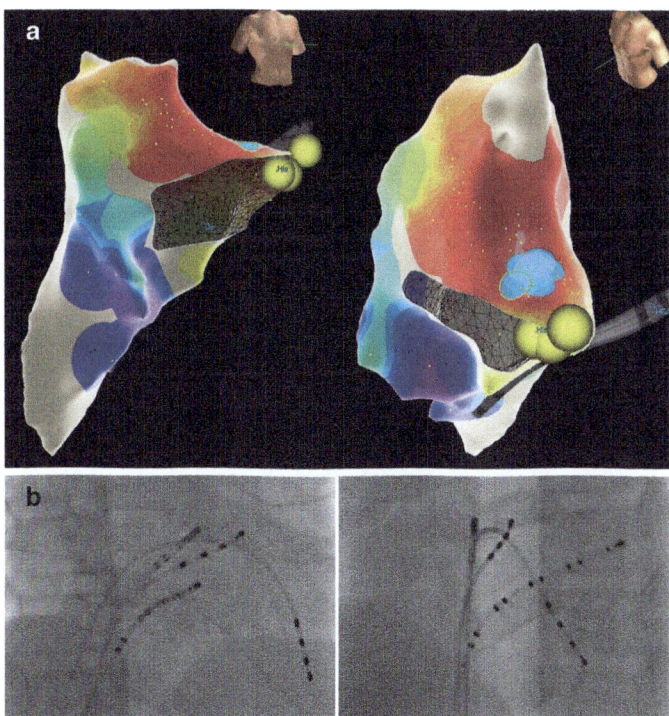

FIGURE 4.10 (**a**) Right atrial activation map (RAO and LAO/cranial views) of earliest atrial activation in AVRT of the patient in Fig. 4.8 with an anteroseptal pathway. *Yellow markers* indicate sites where His potential was recorded; *white/pink* coloration indicates the area of earliest activation; *blue markers* indicate site of successful cryoablation. (**b**) Corresponding fluoroscopy (RAO and LAO views) of catheter positions at the successful site. (**c**) Electrograms from the surface ECG, His, coronary sinus, RV, and ablation catheter at the successful site

diagnostically (e.g. in evaluating whether an SVT is AVRT) or when there is uncertainty about whether the pathway is left-sided or right-sided (although usually this is evident from the retrograde atrial activation sequencing, see Fig. 4.8). When performed, the maneuvers are comparable to those used for AVRT.

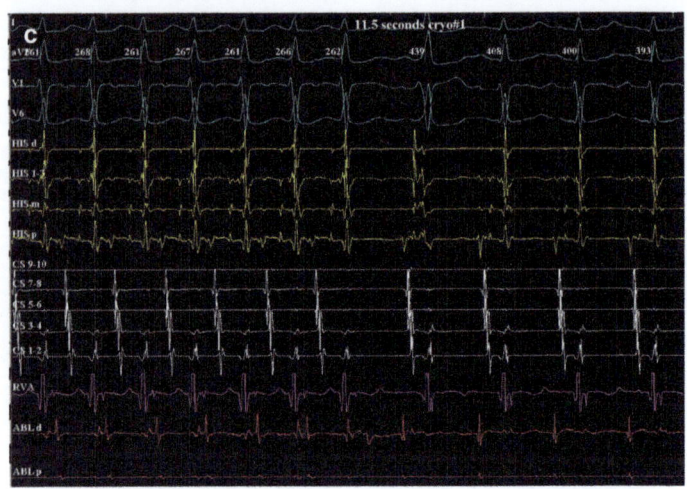

FIGURE 4.10 (continued)

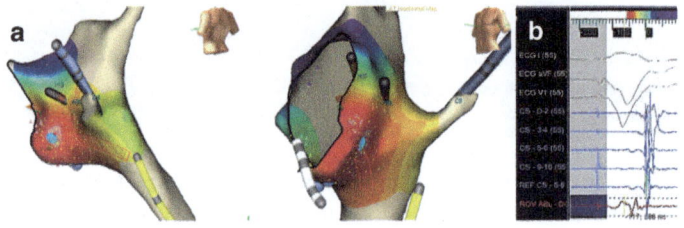

FIGURE 4.11 (**a**) Right atrial activation map (LPO and LAO views) of earliest atrial activation in ventricular pacing of a patient with a right posteroseptal pathway. *White/pink* coloration indicates the area of earliest activation; *blue marker* indicates the site of successful cryoablation. (**b**) Electrograms from the surface ECG, coronary sinus, and roving/ablation catheter at the site indicated by the small *red dot*

Ablation

Correct, precise mapping is the cornerstone of successful WPW ablation. Most pathways are delicate and can be easily eliminated with energy delivery at the correct location. However, there are important considerations with regard to

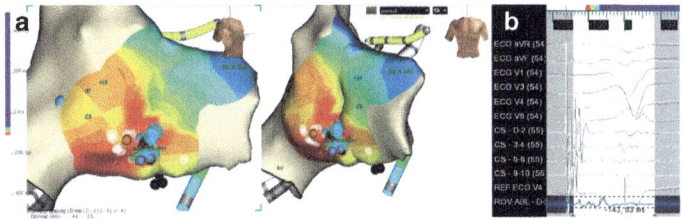

FIGURE 4.12 (**a**) Right ventricular activation map (RAO and AP views) of earliest ventricular activation in atrial pacing of a patient with WPW and three accessory pathways (one right posteroseptal and two right posterolateral). Mapping was quite difficult due to multiple pathways and a prominent Eustachian valve, so several mapping strategies were needed to achieve success. *White/pink* coloration indicates the area of earliest activation during one portion of the study; various color markers indicate sites of interest and/or different ablation lesion sets. The indentation between the atrial and ventricular chambers is somewhat apical of the true annulus. (**b**) Electrograms from the surface ECG, coronary sinus, and roving/ablation catheter near the site of successful ablation

the rhythm in which ablation is performed (see Table 4.1). Because cardiac filling can vary with heartrate and A-V relationship, the exact location of the pathway may differ between different rhythms and therefore ablation is ideally performed in the same rhythm as mapping.

Catheter stability can be an issue with abrupt rhythm changes at the moment of ablation success, such as when AVRT breaks to sinus rhythm. One strategy to minimize this is to map in AVRT, and then ablate in V-entrained AVRT. By carefully entraining just slightly faster than the tachycardia (often achieving sustained fusion in QRS morphology), the map remains accurate, but at the time of pathway success there is only a small change in hemodynamics (from fused tachycardia to fully paced tachycardia) and thus less chance of catheter dislodgement. However, this precludes the possibility of monitoring AV node function during ablation. Conversely, catheter stability is less likely to be an issue when ablating in sinus or paced rhythm, except in the situation of

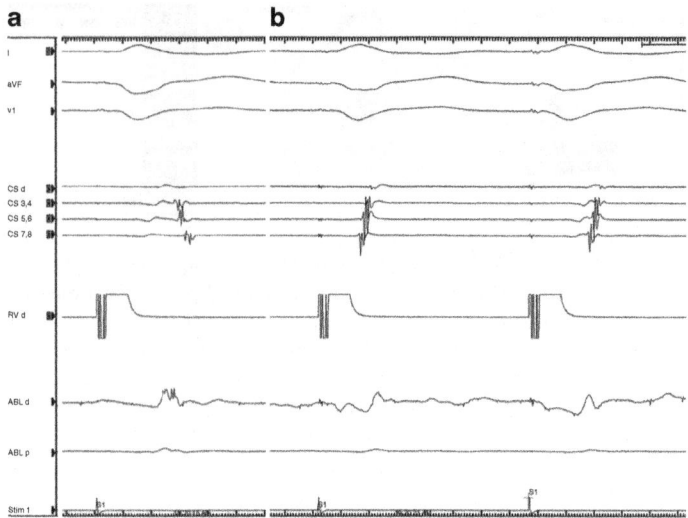

FIGURE 4.13 Surface and intracardiac electrograms (**a**) before and (**b**) just after successful ablation performed during ventricular pacing in a patient with WPW via a left lateral accessory pathway. Note the change from eccentric retrograde conduction (coronary sinus activation distal to proximal) to absent retrograde conduction exposing V-A dissociated sinus rhythm

V paced rhythm with no retrograde nodal conduction, when V-A dissociation can result in canon A waves and intermittent sinus capture beats. (In this situation, quickly switching to simultaneous V and A pacing can improve stability.) Finally, when stability is a persistent issue, cryoablation (with its ability to adhere to tissue) can be helpful even if far from the normal conduction system.

When ablating near the AV node, antegrade properties of the normal conduction system should be continuously monitored. This is easy in orthodromic AVRT (see Fig. 4.10c) as antegrade conduction is exposed during both SVT and sinus rhythm after successful termination. However, it is impossible during ventricular pacing (including V-entrained AVRT), except by alternating between V pacing and A

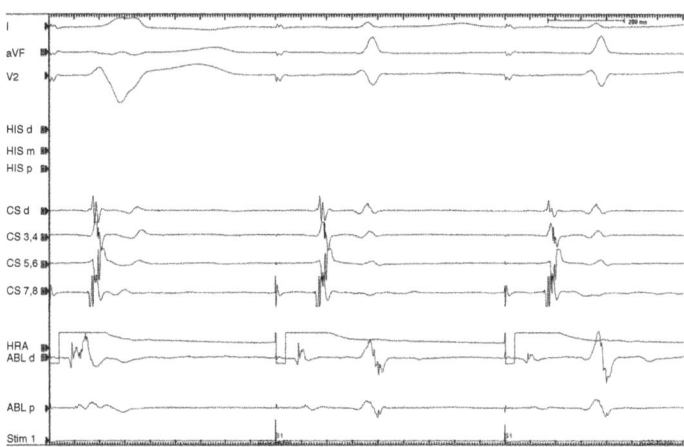

FIGURE 4.14 Surface and intracardiac electrograms showing loss of preexcitation (between first and second beats) due to ablation performed during atrial pacing in a patient with WPW. Note the very early local ventricular activation recorded from the ablation catheter on the first beat, compared to the well-separated atrial and ventricular electrograms on the later beats

pacing in an attempt to monitor both antegrade nodal and retrograde pathway conduction (a technique that is much easier and safer with cryoablation, due to catheter adherence and reversibility of effect). The normal conduction system can also usually be assessed during sinus or atrial paced rhythm, as elimination of both nodal and pathway conduction results in AV block, and elimination of nodal conduction alone results in QRS widening (maximal preexcitation). However, when preexcitation is maximal at baseline (due to rapid atrial pacing, see Fig. 4.1c, or when nodal conduction times are long or the pacing site is much nearer to pathway than node), it is possible to injure the normal conduction without any outward sign. Unfortunately, this results in a tradeoff between optimal mapping (where maximal preexcitation is helpful) and safest ablation (where fused conduction is required).

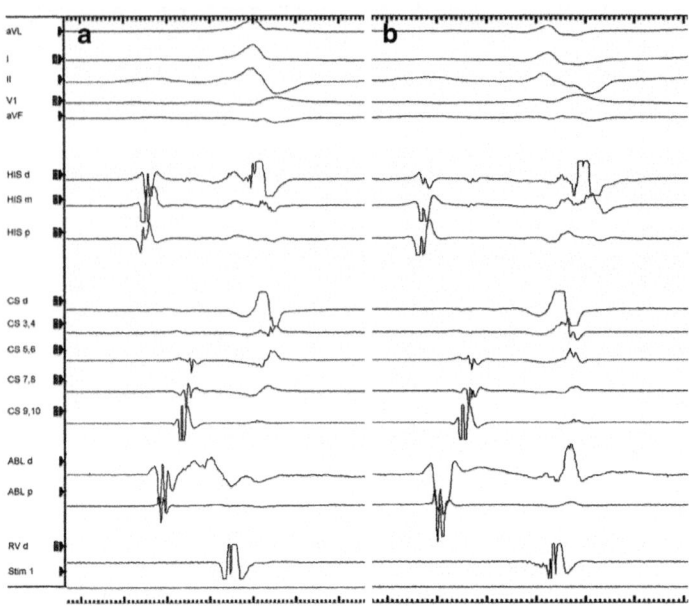

FIGURE 4.15 Surface and intracardiac electrograms (**a**) before and (**b**) just after successful ablation performed during sinus rhythm in a patient with WPW. Note again the very early local ventricular activation recorded from the ablation catheter during preexcitation, compared to the well-separated atrial and ventricular electrograms during nodal conduction. Unlike the previous figure, this patient has relatively subtle preexcitation so the changes in surface PR interval and coronary sinus AV interval are less prominent than the local change at the ablation site

Once a mapping strategy has been chosen and executed, an appropriate site identified, and an ablation strategy selected, the catheter is carefully positioned and energy delivered. It is important to anticipate what aspects of the rhythm need to be watched during ablation (to assess effect, and if necessary to monitor AV node conduction); usually success is obvious (see Figs. 4.13 and 4.14) but occasionally it can be

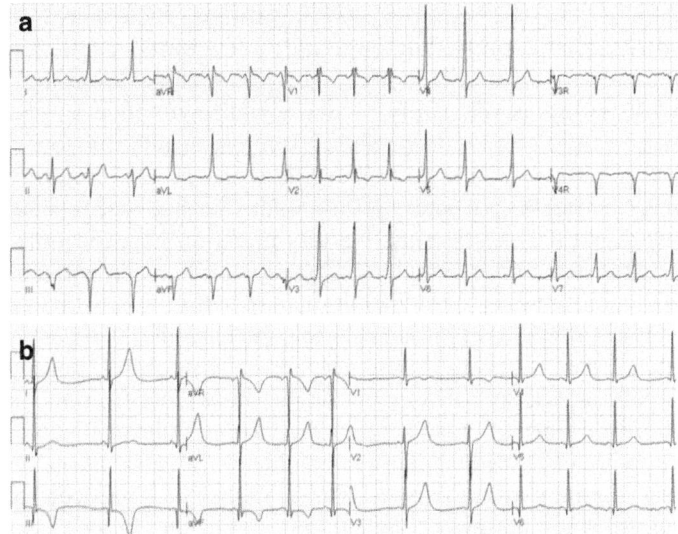

FIGURE 4.16 (**a**) Baseline ECG of a patient with WPW due to a middle cardiac vein pathway. Despite the subtle difference in preexcitation on the first beat, the patient had only one pathway. (**b**) Same patient immediately after ablation, demonstrating repolarization abnormalities consistent with the "T wave memory" phenomenon

fairly subtle (see Fig. 4.15). At an optimal site, pathway conduction can frequently be eliminated within a second or two of RF delivery. Ongoing ablation (beyond 5 or at most 10 s) should be avoided at ineffective sites; although "success" will sometimes be achieved late, this is often due to partial heating from the periphery of the lesion, raising the risk of early recurrence (sometimes immediately after energy delivery is completed, or even during the lesion). Additionally, these lesions can result in tissue edema and local electrogram fragmentation, both of which can interfere with subsequent mapping and ablation. Usually, careful adjustment of the targeted site (with further mapping using the same or a different strategy, if necessary) will ultimately result in a rapidly successful lesion. For the same reasons, large tip or irrigated RF should rarely be required, except perhaps when delivered power is temperature-limited to only a few watts (a situation occasionally encountered with right posteroseptal pathways). Most pathways with early coronary sinus activation can be more safely ablated from within the left atrium, but occasional pathways are truly best targeted in the coronary venous system (particularly the middle cardiac vein), being aware of the risk of coronary artery injury in these locations.

After ablation, a complete EP study should be repeated to document absence of any additional arrhythmia substrate or (if relevant) AV node injury. Of note, patients that had preexcited atrial fibrillation do not typically require therapy beyond accessory pathway ablation (which seems to remove the atrial fibrillation substrate). Adenosine bolus can sometimes unmask residual pathway conduction, and is reasonable as a routine part of the post-ablation study, but is particularly helpful when pathway conduction is absent due to mechanical trauma or edema from an imperfectly targeted ablation attempt. Post-ablation repolarization abnormalities, including T wave inversion and QT prolongation, are quite common after WPW ablation and attributed to "T wave memory" or "cardiac memory" (see Fig. 4.16); frank ST depression or elevation is less common and should prompt consideration of coronary artery injury. A 30–60 min waiting period is prudent because of the chance of early recurrence.

Reference

1. Pediatric and Congenital Electrophysiology Society (PACES); Heart Rhythm Society (HRS); American College of Cardiology Foundation (ACCF); American Heart Association (AHA); American Academy of Pediatrics (AAP); Canadian Heart Rhythm Society (CHRS), Cohen MI, Triedman JK, Cannon BC, Davis AM, Drago F, Janousek J, Klein GJ, Law IH, Morady FJ, Paul T, Perry JC, Sanatani S, Tanel RE. PACES/HRS expert consensus statement on the management of the asymptomatic young patient with a Wolff-Parkinson-White (WPW, ventricular preexcitation) electrocardiographic pattern: developed in partnership between the

Pediatric and Congenital Electrophysiology Society (PACES) and the Heart Rhythm Society (HRS). Endorsed by the governing bodies of PACES, HRS, the American College of Cardiology Foundation (ACCF), the American Heart Association (AHA), the American Academy of Pediatrics (AAP), and the Canadian Heart Rhythm Society (CHRS). Heart Rhythm. 2012;9(6):1006–24. doi:10.1016/j.hrthm.2012.03.050. Epub 2012 May 10.

Chapter 5
Atrial Flutter

David T. Huang and Travis Prinzi

Atrial flutter is a macroreentrant tachycardia. It is most commonly found in its typical form in which the reentrant circuit travels around the right atrium in a counterclockwise and sometimes clockwise fashion. Atrial flutter can also be a more complex arrhythmia, traveling around scars or other lines of block in either the right or left atrium; these "atypical flutters" are also referred to as macrooreentrant atrial tachycardias.

Incidence and Etiologies

The incidence of atrial flutter is largely unknown due to a lack of organized data in the general population. Most of the epidemiologic data on atrial flutter have been grouped together with data from patients with atrial fibrillation. The estimate for the incidence of new cases of atrial flutter in the United States is around 200,000 per year.

D.T. Huang, MD (✉) • T. Prinzi, MD
Department of Cardiology, University of Rochester
Medical Center, Rochester, NY, USA
e-mail: David_Huang@URMC.Rochester.edu

D.T. Huang, T. Prinzi (eds.), *Clinical Cardiac*
Electrophysiology in Clinical Practice, In Clinical Practice,
DOI 10.1007/978-1-4471-5433-4_5,
© Springer-Verlag London 2015

As with atrial fibrillation, atrial flutter occurs more frequently in patients with structural heart disease. Although the causes of atrial flutter are not entirely understood, certain conditions have been implicated or associated with a higher risk for developing atrial flutter. These include hypertension, coronary artery disease, congestive heart failure and valvular heart disease such as those resulting from rheumatic heart disease [1]. It is thought that any condition that leads to an increased stretch and load on the atria can be a potential cause for any atrial arrhythmia. Congenital heart disease, either surgically repaired or not, and cardiac surgery, either involving an incision in the atrium or not, are also common causes of atrial flutter. Other conditions such as an overactive thyroid, fever, lung disease, or even alcohol can be associated with atrial flutter. Many of these mechanisms are still not well delineated, although it appears that inflammation may play a role in the pathogenesis.

Classification

Atrial flutter has been classified several ways. Historically, it has been described as "typical" vs. "atypical," initially based on the rate of the flutter in the atrium and with the most commonly encountered variant termed as "typical" flutter [2]. In 2001, the North American Society of Pacing and Electrophysiology proposed a different classification system based on mechanism of the flutter as well as the anatomic circuits involved [3]. "Typical" or "Type I" atrial flutter displays a classic pattern of downward deflecting "saw-tooth" flutter waves on the inferior leads of 12 lead EKG and the flutter waves are of a positive polarity (upright) in the early precordial leads, V1 and V2 (see Fig. 5.1). By convention, "Atypical" or "Type II" atrial flutter are those that display any other patterns on the 12 lead EKG.

Mechanisms of Atrial Flutter

Atrial flutter can best be distinguished from atrial tachycardia in that atrial flutter is a reentrant circuit, whereas atrial tachycardia is focal. During atrial flutter, the electrical signal

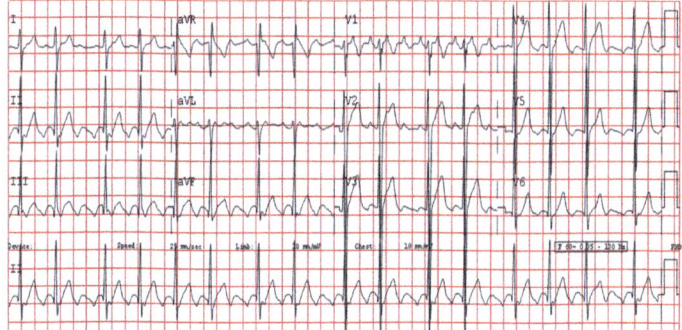

FIGURE 5.1 Typical atrial flutter EKG. Notice classic "saw tooth" p waves in inferior leads, and positive p waves in V1 and V2

in the atrium traverses around in a fixed circuit. The circuit can involve the entire right or left atrium or just part(s) of the atrium. In contrast, an atrial tachycardia originates from a focal source in the atrium, i.e., a group of cells firing off abnormal electrical activity. Atrial flutter can be distinguished from atrial fibrillation (AF) by the organization of the flutter circuit within the atria. The circuit leading to atrial flutter often is well organized, meaning that the path of the circuit is the same with each flutter cycle length, and it repeats itself over and over again. Occasionally, atrial flutter can involve more than one stable circuit. Atrial flutter is distinguished from AF in that AF is a much more disorganized atrial arrhythmia. There is no stable circuit in fibrillation. In AF, the signals in the atria are often crashing into themselves or into each other.

In order for a reentering impulse to be continually repetitive as in "Typical" or "Type I" atrial flutter, it needs to be a stable circuit. The stability of the circuit is attributed to the presence of an excitable gap, where the heart tissue trailing the traversing impulse has recovered from refractoriness and is able to be excited again. In addition, there is an area of slow conduction within the circuit. These conditions fulfill the two requirements for impulse reentry (1. different impulse travel speeds or conduction velocities in two pathways where the electrical signals can go through; 2.

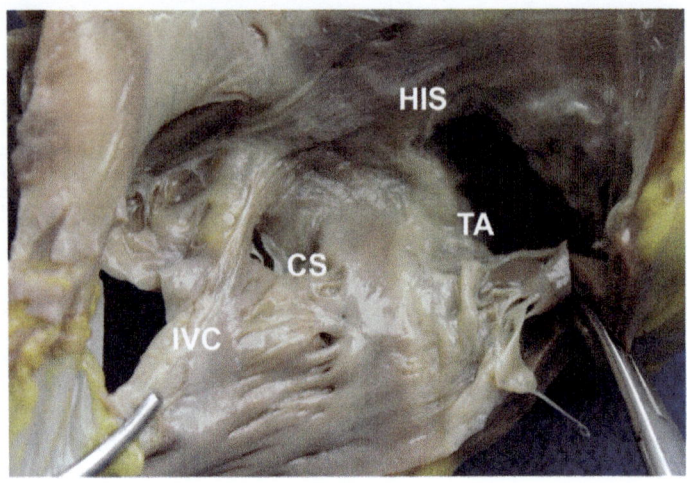

FIGURE 5.2 RA anatomy for typical atrial flutter. *IVC* inferior vena cava, *CS* coronary sinus, *TA* tricuspid annulus, *His* bundle of His

differential refractoriness of the tissues in these two pathways). The areas of slow conduction can be a result of anatomic variations (variable patterns in cell alignment, the so called "anisotropy", or anatomic structures that are more fibrous and less conducting) or as a result of scar from inflammation, surgery or stretch. In patients who present with the most commonly encountered atrial flutter ("typical atrial flutter"), this area of slow conduction coincides with the region between the tricuspid valve and the inferior vena cava and bordered by the Eustachian ridge (see Fig. 5.2). This is often referred to as the "cavo-tricuspid isthmus" because it forms a bridge of tissue through which the circuit is sustained. These slow conduction areas often become targets for ablation where if the reentering circuit can be interrupted or cut permanently, then the atrial flutter can be considered cured. This can be achieved with ablation through the circuit resulting in complete conduction block across the isthmus.

The traditional classification of "Atypical" or "Type II" atrial flutter had involved circuits other than the one traveling through the cavo-tricuspid isthmus. With better mapping techniques and improved understanding, these "atypical" atrial flutters have now been defined further. Atypical atrial flutter can involve either the right or the left atrium. It is now well know that ablations in the left atrium, particularly for atrial fibrillation, can result in atrial flutter as an unintended outcome of the ablation procedure. During an ablation for AF, linear ablation lesions create barriers in the left atrium to isolate the areas where fibrillation originates. These barriers, if not contiguous, can have gaps in the line or create areas of slow conduction. This can in turn set up conditions needed for flutter circuits in the left atrium. Some of more commonly encountered circuits, the "roof-dependent" flutters, involve circuits traveling around the right or left pulmonary veins (Fig. 5.3). Another commonly occurring atrial flutter travels around the mitral annulus using the gap between the left inferior pulmonary vein and the mitral annulus (or the so-called left atrial isthmus) (Fig. 5.4).

Scarring from inflammation, surgery or ischemia/infarct can also create conditions leading to barriers within the atrial tissue that, in turn, set up the atrium for flutter circuits. Complex circuits have been mapped and reported which lead to another variant of "atypical" atrial flutter. Most atrial flutters involve a single circuit, but there may be multiple circuits involved. One such two-circuit or "dual-loop" example that has been reported involves one circuit that participates in a "typical flutter" fashion, going through the cavo-tricuspid isthmus, and at the same time a secondary circuit going through a scar area on the more lateral aspect of the right atrium. These circuits traverse through the atrium together in a "figure of 8" pattern, facilitating and sustaining one another (Fig. 5.5, Media 3–4). When multiple circuits are involved, there often is a coordinated activation around these circuits, meaning that the signals travel through these circuits at a fixed rate from beat to beat, thus creating a stable flutter. For these more complex flutters, ablation may be needed across

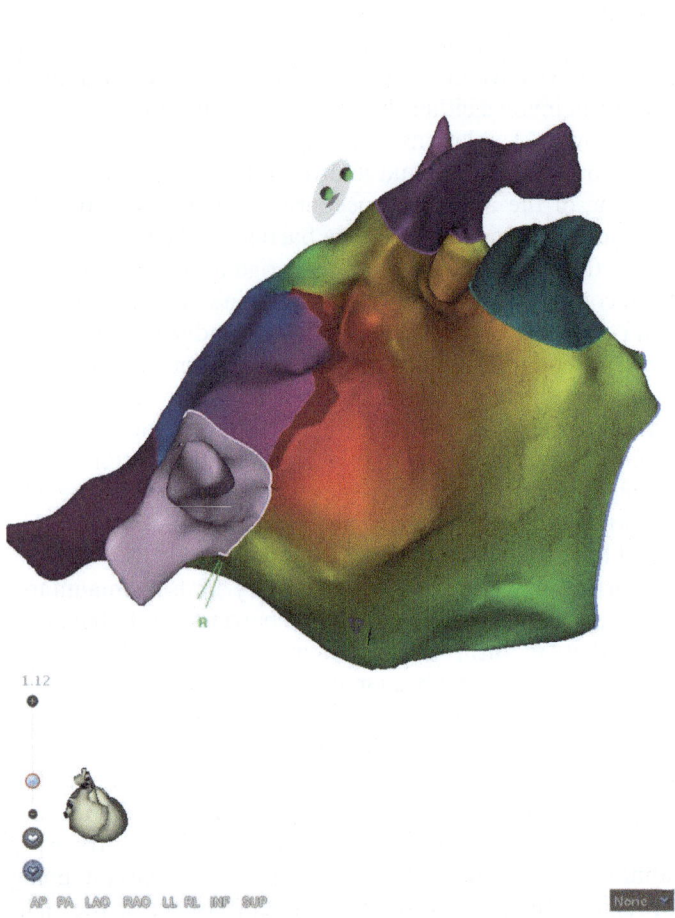

FIGURE 5.3 Roof-dependent left atrial flutter. "Early meets late" on the roof near the right veins

multiple circuits in order to terminate the atrial flutter and convert to normal sinus rhythm, as well as to prevent further recurrences of signals traveling around either one of the circuits.

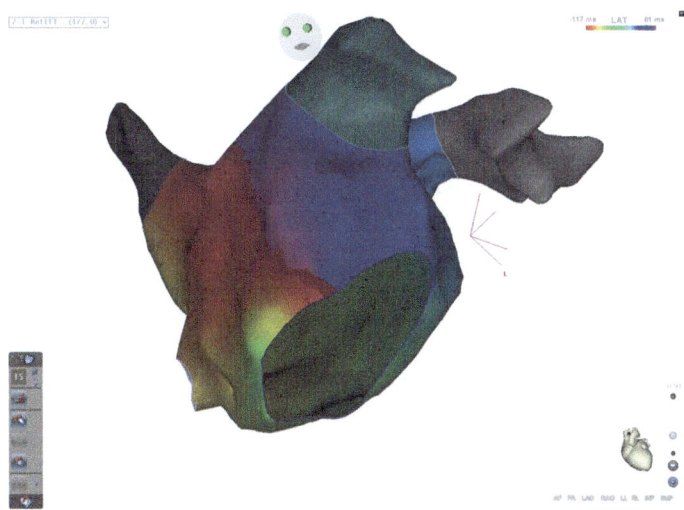

FIGURE 5.4 Mitral Isthmus flutter. The entire cycle length of the tachycardia can be found around the mitral annulus

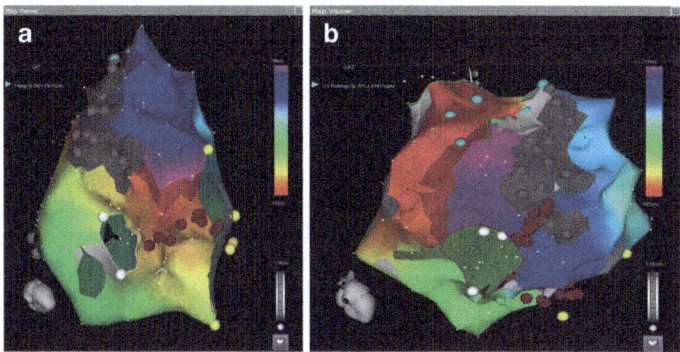

FIGURE 5.5 (**a**) Typical flutter circuit of dual loop flutter, traveling around CTI. (**b**) Secondary circuit of dual loop flutter, traveling around RA lateral wall scar

Management

Many options are available for the treatment of atrial flutter, and treatment should be tailored to individual patient needs and circumstances. These can range from cautious monitoring to invasive therapy with catheter ablation. As atrial flutter is a non-life-threatening arrhythmic condition, symptomatic control is often the primary goal for therapy. Other important reasons for treating atrial flutter also include reducing the risk of tachycardia-mediated cardiomyopathy and minimizing recurrent heart failure exacerbation.

In general, the goals in managing atrial flutter include: control of ventricular rates during atrial flutter, restoration of regular sinus rhythm, and prevention of thromboembolic events. A wide variety of drugs can be utilized for medical therapy, such as beta blockers or calcium channel blockers that control the ventricular response rate, membrane active antiarrhythmic drugs such as propafenone, flecainide or ibutilide to restore sinus rhythm, and anticoagulants such as warfarin or dabigatran to reduce the risks of embolic events such as stroke.

Catheter based therapy has now become accepted as another first line treatment for patients with atrial flutter, especially ones with "typical" or "type I" variant. It offers a potential curative option and much improved long-term maintenance of sinus rhythm as compared with medical therapy [4]. The technical aspects of ablation have been discussed in section "Technical considerations". The primary aim in ablation for atrial flutter is to interrupt the reentrant circuit permanently. Thus the main strategy in mapping atrial flutter is to locate an isthmus (narrow ridge) of tissue where the electrical impulse in the atrium travels through two electrically inactive boundary areas, such as anatomical structures like the tricuspid valve and the inferior vena cava, or scars. The goal of the ablation needs to be more than the restoration of sinus mechanism. To achieve electrical conduction block across the critical isthmus of the flutter circuit completely is regarded as the successful endpoint. It's important not only that the arrhythmia stop, but that it can never come back.

In patients with atypical flutter that is refractory to conventional curative ablation and medical therapy, ablation of the atrioventricular node is another strategy that can be used to treat patients with atrial flutter. This ablation will induce significant bradycardia, and a pacemaker will be needed to maintain an adequate heart rate. Pacing usually involves single right ventricular lead stimulation. Alternatively, biventricular pacing devices have been used which may improve long term hemodynamic response in patients and lower incidence of heart failure.

Prevention of thromboembolic events with anticoagulation therapy is another main objective in the treatment of patients with atrial flutter. For patients assessed to be at risk, such as those with heart failure, structural heart disease, older age, and prior stroke or transient ischemic attacks, therapy with anticoagulants is recommended. Warfarin has been a mainstay medication traditionally. Newer antithrombin agents such as dabigatran and rivaroxaban have been demonstrated to be effective alternatives.

Technical Considerations

Mapping

The best way to assess atrial flutter and macro-reentrant atrial tachyarrhythmias is by careful and thorough 3-dimensional mapping. The first step is to choose a consistent reference to be "time zero" for the activation map, a fixed location of electrical activation. This needs to be from a catheter that will reliably stay in the same anatomic position recording electrical signals timed consistently with every cycle, so that "time zero" never changes. Usually, the best catheter to use as a reference is a bipolar electrogram (EGM) on the coronary sinus catheter, which should stay in place throughout the entire procedure and sits epicardially to the LA, so is less prone to movement during the manipulation of the mapping catheter. The mapping catheter is manipulated

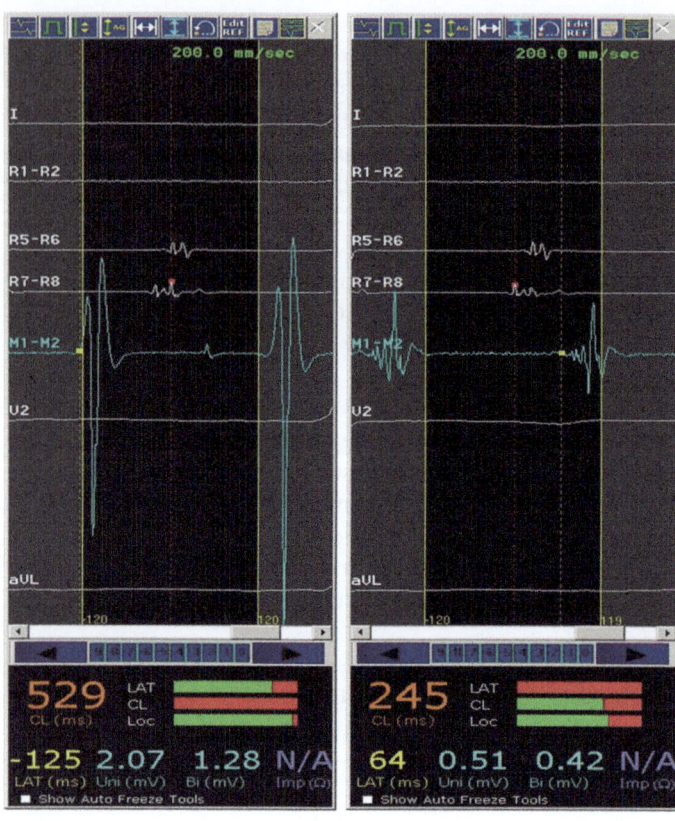

FIGURE 5.6 Note the shifted reference. R7-R8 is fractionated. In the first point, the later part of the EGM is tagged. In the second point, the earlier component is tagged. This will distort your map, as seen in Fig. 5.7

by the operator in the chamber of interest. In atrial flutters, it roves around the atria gathering local electrical activation (EA) data. Be certain to choose a sharp and reliable EGM. Fractionated EGMs can cause a distortion of data, because "time zero" shifts to different places along the fractionated EGM (see Figs. 5.5a, b and 5.6a, b, Media 3–4). As the catheter is manipulated around the atrium, points are

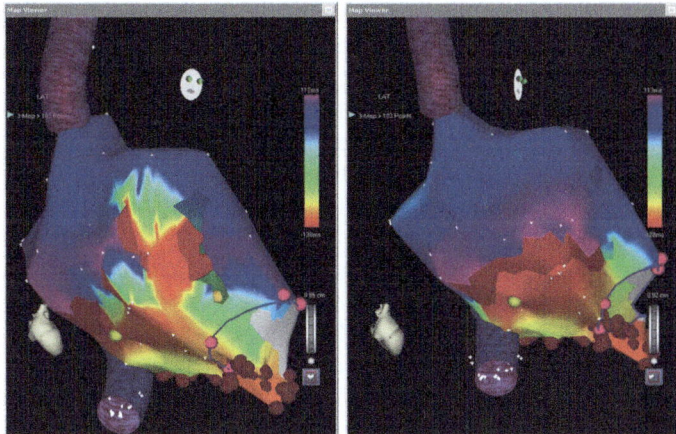

FIGURE 5.7 The map on the *left* is confusing, with no clear early-meets-late, because of a shifting reference throughout procedure. The map on the *right* is the exact same case, corrected, with careful attention to the reference being selected on the same part of the EGM. There is a clear early-meets-late, and typical atrial flutter is confirmed (See Media 5–6 for propagation of these two maps)

collected on the mapping system when the physician confirms he or she has contact with the endocardium, and the point is annotated to the first sharp deflection on the bipolar EGM (confirm with first sharp down stroke of unipolar EGM to rule out far field atrial signal).

Once a reliable reference is chosen, the next step is to set the window of interest (WOI) for activation mapping. Traditionally, local activation time (LAT) mapping for macro-reentrant arrhythmias has been done by calculating 90 % of the tachycardia cycle length (TCL), and splitting that number 50/50 on either side of the reference EGM. So if the TCL is 220 ms, the window will be 199 ms, with 98 ms on either side of the reference EGM. So the WOI would be −98 ms to 98 ms. This is a quick method of setting the WOI, and mapping 90 % will demonstrate, if the operator is mapping a reentrant circuit and is doing so in the correct chamber, a transition area where the earliest measured signal meets up with the latest measured signal ("early-meets-late"). This helps to confirm that the arrhythmia is indeed originating in the particular chamber mapped, and the details of the impulse circuit demonstrate where the reentrant circuit is traveling.

There, however, are cons to using this method. Because LAT data is collected in reference to an arbitrary "time zero," the "early-meets-late" is also arbitrary. It shows *that* the arrhythmia is reentrant and *where* the circuit is traveling, but it does not serve as a guide for where to ablate. In other words, ablating along the early-meets-late line on the mapping system will not necessarily terminate the arrhythmia. For typical atrial flutter, this hardly matters. In typical atrial flutter, the shortest line between two electrically isolated structures is the cavo-tricuspid isthmus (the ridge of tissue separated by the boundaries of inferior vena cava and the tricuspid valve), and this is what will be regularly targeted for ablation (more on this below).

If, however, the tachycardia is somewhere in the left atrium, or traveling around a scar in either atrium, deciding on a target for curative ablation can be trickier. While the standard 90 % TCL, 50/50 window will give the basic data for the reentrant circuit, a more advanced but beneficial algorithm for setting the WOI may be used. Robert DePonti has proposed the following for setting the mapping window: Using this method, the early-meets-late line on the 3D map will be placed in the circuit's mid-diastolic isthmus (MDI), the zone of slow conduction [5]. In atypical flutters that are less clear, mapping the mid-diastolic isthmus provides a more helpful picture of the tachycardia circuit and may also guide ablation, as the MDI for atypical flutter is usually found in low voltage and scar areas.

$$\text{Backward interval} = (\text{TCL} - \text{Pwave duration}) / 2$$
$$+ \text{Interval}: \text{PwaveOnset} \quad \text{REF}$$
$$\text{Forward interval} = (\text{TCL} - \text{Backward interval}) \times .9$$

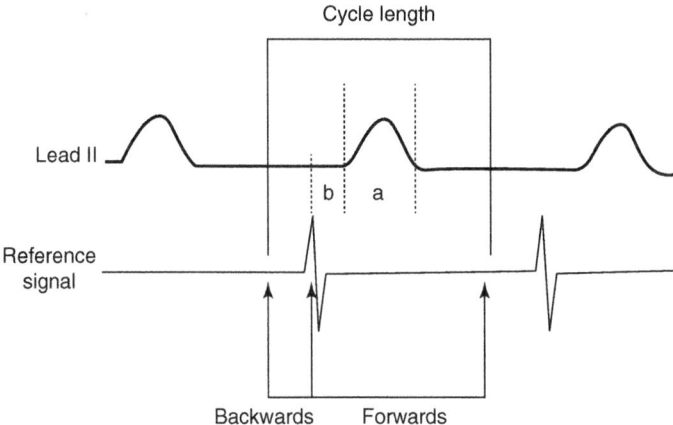

To make it less complicated, the basic concept is to put the P wave in the middle of the window, and to put the "early meets late" portion of the cycle length in the middle of atrial diastole (between two P waves).

Entrainment

Pacing during any arrhythmia can also aid in the mapping of the electrical circuit. In a reentrant circuit, pacing and the response of the local activation where pacing is taking place can help one locate the critical isthmus of the circuit. The pacing is performed from the selected site at a rate that is slightly faster than the native flutter rate (about 10–15 % faster). The pacing site will only capture if pacing is occurring at a faster rate than the native rate. If pacing takes place within an area the circuit traverses through, the first post pacing cycle length ("post pacing interval") should equal to the native flutter cycle length (give or take 10 % to permit for conduction delay associated with faster pacing rates and measurement errors). Furthermore, if this is combined with concealed entrainment – if the flutter wave morphology on the surface ECG is the identical to the paced p wave or atrial deflection on the surface ECG – then one can be assured that the pacing site is a part of the circuit. This circuit should then be the target of ablation. If the isthmus comprises a small region, a point lesion may suffice in terminating the arrhythmia. On the other hand, if the region is relatively larger in size, as in most flutters, a linear ablation across boundaries of this area, such as the tricuspid valve and the inferior vena cava for "typical" atrial flutter, is needed to terminate the arrhythmia and to prevent any further arrhythmia recurrence through the same circuit and the same isthmus. If the surface ECG atrial waves exhibit a different morphology than during the native flutter, then the pacing is called a manifest or non-concealed entrainment. This site is not part of the circuit and ablation in this area will not be successful in terminating the arrhythmia.

Ablation

The goal of ablation therapy for an arrhythmia involving a reentrant mechanism is to interrupt the circuit permanently so that normal sinus rhythm can be restored and the recurrence of the same arrhythmia can be prevented. Strategies for ablation often target between two electrically inactive structures bordering an area that is critical to the reentrant circuit (called a "critical isthmus" part of the circuit) and to create a line of electrical block in this region. This can cut through the path of the circuit and by taking advantage of the surrounding anatomic structures that do not conduct electrical signals, the barriers to conduction will no longer permit the electrical impulses to reenter leading to a recurrence of the same arrhythmia.

In typical atrial flutter, this ablation is performed at the cavo-tricuspid isthmus (see Fig. 5.2). It is well known that the typical flutter circuit travels through the area between the tricuspid valve and the inferior vena cava. By cutting the conduction through this isthmus region, the electrical impulse cannot travel through this and the surrounding tricuspid valve and the inferior vena cava the flutter can be cured. Other areas in the right atrium may potentially be targeted for ablation but these may be impractical because of the larger areas involved and/or proximity to sensitive functional structures such as the sinoatrial or the atrioventricular nodes. The cavo-tricuspid isthmus is readily accessible through an inferior venous approach from the femoral vein and does not contain vital structures to the function of the heart. Therefore, it is an ideal region to target for ablation. In "atypical" atrial flutter, linear lesions are often created between scars, or between a previous ablation line and another electrically isolated structure (e.g., lateral wall right atrial scar to inferior vena cava, or left inferior pulmonary vein isolation line to mitral valve).

Several catheter options and modalities are available for the creation of a linear lesion, including longer-tip radiofrequency ablation catheters (8 mm or 10 mm), irrigated-tip radiofrequency ablation, or cryoablation. Settings (power-controlled or temperature-controlled) will depend on catheter choice and area being treated.

Where to ablate across the cavo-tricuspid isthmus for typical flutter is an important consideration. The shortest distance across the isthmus is around 6 o'clock on the tricuspid annulus, based on a left anterior oblique projection of the heart. The anatomy there is prone, however, to be associated with diverticulum, or "pouches", in the tissue, making it more difficult to drag an ablation line. A more medial approach (5 o'clock on the same projection) may also have pouches, and it is closer to sensitive structures like the coronary sinus ostium and the atrioventricular node. A lateral approach (7 o'clock) allows you to avoid pouches, but the atrial musculature tends to be thicker and pectinate muscles may also be located here, leading to a lower likelihood of successful transmural ablation lesions. Each patient may have variations on these issues and anatomic along with electrical voltage mapping of the area targeted for ablation can be helpful in selecting the best suitable site for ablation therapy.

When dealing with atypical flutters, determining location for a line of block can be more difficult. In the case of mitral isthmus flutters in the LA, a line is often drawn from a previous left inferior pulmonary vein circumferential isolation line (from an atrial fibrillation ablation) down to the mitral annulus. This area has now been termed as the "left atrial mitral isthmus". Due to the prominence of post-AF ablation atrial flutters observed, electrophysiologists now avoid creating these ablation lines as part of the atrial fibrillation ablation strategy. Nevertheless, these flutters can be observed and is one of the more common atypical atrial flutters that can occur after an atrial fibrillation ablation. Once this type of flutter has been noted to occur spontaneously, the recurrence rate is high and the flutter can often be very persistent leading to more symptoms than the paroxysmal atrial fibrillation. Ablation in the left atrial mitral isthmus region is then needed to eliminate the substrate for this flutter. These ablation lines are notoriously difficult to achieve complete conduction block endocardially within the left atrium and sometimes need to be finished epicardially by ablating within the distal coronary sinus. In the case of LA roof-dependent flutter, linear ablation across roof is created from the right superior pulmonary vein to the left superior pulmonary vein. In the case of scar-mediated atrial flutters, ablation is performed either between two dense scars, or a scar and another electrically isolated structure (see Fig. 5.5 for a right lateral scar to IVC ablation line).

Validation

Successful ablation occurs when bi-directional block is created across a critical isthmus, eliminating the reentering circuit entirely. In typical flutter, this line of block is created between the tricuspid valve and the inferior vena cava. If ablation is performed during atrial flutter, the first step in observing success is the restoration of sinus rhythm. This does not necessarily mean it's time to stop ablating. While the atrial flutter has terminated, one must be certain that no atrial flutter can ever travel through that isthmus again.

There are a few options for confirming bi-directional block across the isthmus. If a Halo catheter has been placed around the tricuspid annulus, or any other kind of 10- or 20-pole catheter has been placed on the lateral wall of the RA, pacing

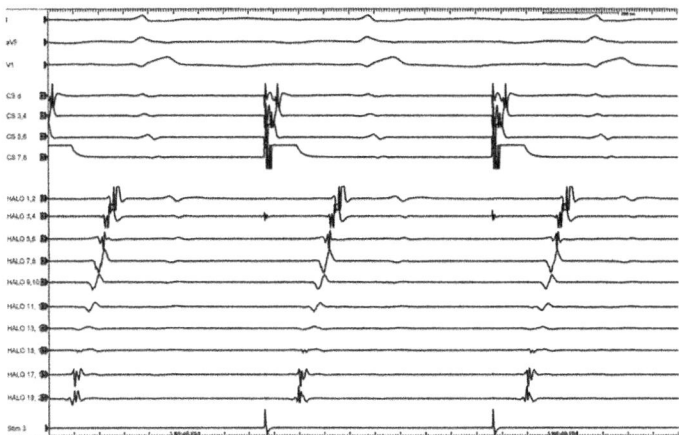

FIGURE 5.8 Pacing from CS, Halo activation is proximal to distal. This means the CTI is blocked

from the coronary sinus will show a proximal-to-distal activation sequence on the Halo (see Fig. 5.8). Pacing in the other direction (from the distal pole of the Halo) will reveal a pattern in which the CS proximal poles will be later than all the poles of the Halo catheter. If, during CS pacing, there is a curved or "Chevron" activation pattern recorded by the Halo catheter (see Fig. 5.9), CTI block is not complete, and more ablation must be done.

For physicians who do not prefer to have an extra catheter in the heart (Halo or other lateral wall catheter) and would rather use a two-catheter approach (CS catheter and ablation), conduction time can be measured to demonstrate block by placing the ablation catheter on the lateral side of the ablation line. The ablation catheter can be placed on the ablation line to look for double potentials while CS pacing. Double potentials that are separated by at least 90 ms are suggestive of CTI block, and if separation is measured to be >115 ms, it can be used to confirm bidirectional block.[1]

---

[1] Morady paper from *JACC*.

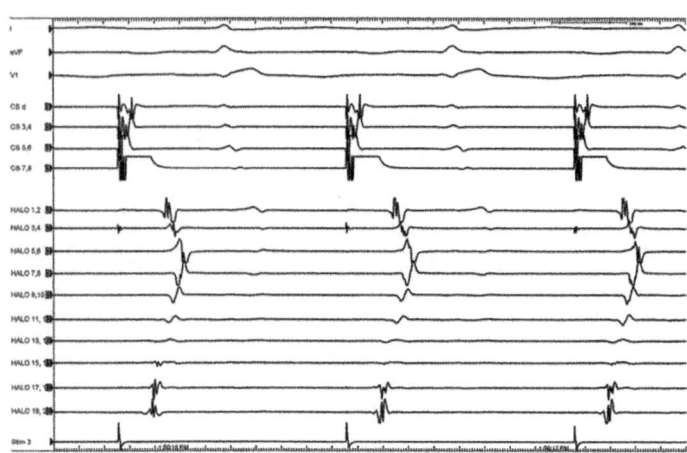

FIGURE 5.9 Pacing from CS catheter, activation on Halo is not proximal to distal. This means activation is still passing through the CTI

A 3 dimensional activation map can be used as another method to validate CTI block, and it is also valuable for assessing the breakthrough point, or conduction gap, if block is not complete. Pacing from CS proximal, with the paced catheter as the "time zero" reference (with a window of approximate +20 to +200), an electroanatomic map should show a clear block of conduction along the ablation line (See Media 7). If block is not present, careful and detailed activation mapping along the ablation line should show where electrical activity is still sneaking through the line of block, and this can serve as a guide to finish ablation. The voltage map of the region can be used to observe where tissue along the line is still active with a substantial voltage mapped and serve as another guide to complete the ablation.

Validation can be more complex with atypical flutter ablation lines, but applying the same principle used in the criteria for typical flutter ablation can be adopted to demonstrate bidirectional block across the associated critical isthmus in atypical flutter cases. By placing catheters on either side of the created line of block and pacing in both directions, bidirectional block across the linear lesion can be confirmed with these additional activation maps.

References

1. Granada J, Uribe W, Chyou PH, Maassen K, Vierkant R, Smith PN, Hayes J, Eaker E, Vidaillet H. Incidence and predictors of atrial flutter in the general population. J Am Coll Cardiol. 2000; 36(7):2242.
2. Wells Jr JL, MacLean WA, James TN, Waldo AL. Characterization of atrial flutter. Studies in man after open heart surgery using fixed atrial electrodes. Circulation. 1979;60:665.
3. Saoudi N, Cosio F, Waldo A, et al. A classification of atrial flutter and regular atrial tachycardia according to electrophysiological mechanisms and anatomic bases; a Statement from a Joint Expert Group from The Working Group of Arrhythmias of the European Society of Cardiology and the North American Society of Pacing and Electrophysiology. Eur Heart J. 2001;22:1162.
4. Natale A, Newby KH, Pisano E, et al. Prospective randomized comparison of antiarrhythmic therapy versus first-line radiofrequency ablation in patients with atrial flutter J Am Coll Cardiol. 2000;35(7):1898–1904.
5. DePonti R. Treatment of macro-re-entrant atrial tachycardia based on electroanatomic mapping: identification and ablation of the mis-diastolic isthmus. Eurospace. 2007;9:449–57.

Chapter 6
A Practical Guide to Radiofrequency Catheter Ablation of Atrial Fibrillation

Burr W. Hall and Travis Prinzi

Introduction

Atrial fibrillation (AF) continues to be the most common cardiac rhythm disturbance encountered in clinical practice. It is estimated that greater than 2.2 million people in the United States are affected by AF with a prevalence reaching 0.4–1 % of the general population [1–3]. Hospitalizations for AF have also significantly increased due to an increase in the prevalence of chronic heart disease, an increase in the ageing population, and an increase in detection by ambulatory monitoring [4–6]. The clinical consequences of AF range from diminished quality of life and increase in congestive heart failure, to devastating thromboembolic events and increased mortality [7–10].

Treatment of AF has long been achieved with maintenance of sinus rhythm or managing heart rate with pharmacologic agents [2, 11]. Over the past decade, radiofrequency catheter ablation (RFCA) has been offered as an alternative

B.W. Hall, MD (✉)
Department of Cardiology, Atrial Fibrillation Clinic,
University of Rochester Medical Center, Rochester, NY, USA
e-mail: Burr_Hall@urmc.rochester.edu

T. Prinzi, MD
Department of Cardiology, University of Rochester
Medical Center, Rochester, NY, USA

D.T. Huang, T. Prinzi (eds.), *Clinical Cardiac
Electrophysiology in Clinical Practice*, In Clinical Practice,
DOI 10.1007/978-1-4471-5433-4_6,
© Springer-Verlag London 2015

99

or in conjunction with medical therapy in patients either with refractory AF or with intolerance to antiarrhythmic medications. With improvements in technique and skill, RFCA has provided an important alternative for specific patient populations in whom AF is refractory to antiarrhythmic medications. Despite advances in ablation therapy, AF recurrences are common and the number of patients requiring repeat procedures is not insignificant. AF ablation success rates have varied between centers with reported procedural success rates between 68 and 86 % at 1 year [12, 13]. Although AF ablation is now performed worldwide, its proper place in the treatment algorithms remains subject to debate despite being included within the most recent ACC AHA guidelines [14].

In this chapter we describe how we have been performing RFCA of AF over the past decade at the University of Rochester Medical Center. While AF ablation technique may vary across medical institutions, we share our protocol as we have found that the methods that we describe have served us very well from both a safety and efficacy standpoint.

Patient Selection

The primary indication for ablation of AF should be to improve arrhythmia related symptoms such as palpitations, fatigue, shortness of breath and exercise intolerance. There is little to no data to suggest that AF ablation can reduce mortality and therefore symptom improvement should be the primary goal of AF ablation. We have seen patients in our practice with asymptomatic AF who are interested in proceeding with AF ablation as an alternative to long-term systemic anticoagulation. While there is limited data demonstrating that discontinuation of warfarin post AF ablation is safe in the short to medium term follow-up in specific patient populations, this has not been confirmed by larger randomized clinical trials [15–17]. It has therefore always been our practice not to discontinue warfarin or equivalent therapies post-ablation in patients that have a high risk of stroke as determined by the CHA2Ds2-VASC score regardless of the presence or absence of AF.

Consensus indications for RFCA of AF have been well described in the 2012 HRS/EHRA/ECAS expert consensus statement [18]. While these guidelines are very helpful in determining the appropriateness of AF ablation in a specific patient cohort, it is also imperative that patient preference be carefully considered. AF ablation is a complex procedure with procedural risk and the risk benefit ratio of performing such a procedure must be carefully considered for each patient. There are many clinical and imaging based variables that can be used to help define the efficacy and procedural risk of AF ablation in an individual patient which are summarized in Table 6.1.

In our own experience we have found that left atrial volume is the predominant predictor of AF ablation success. In a subset of 88 patients with both paroxysmal and persistent

TABLE 6.1 Patient selection for AF ablation

Patient characteristic	Better candidate	Worse candidate
Symptoms	Highly symptomatic	Asymptomatic
Failed Class I or III antiarrhythmic drugs	>1	0
AF classification	Paroxysmal	Long standing persistent
Age at time of ablation	Younger (<70)	Older (>70)
Left atrial size	<80 cc	>120 cc
Ejection fraction	Normal	Reduced
CHF	No	Yes
Concomitant cardiac disease	No	Yes
Pulmonary disease	No	Yes
Obstructive sleep apnea	No	Yes
Obesity	No	Yes
Prior stroke	No	Yes

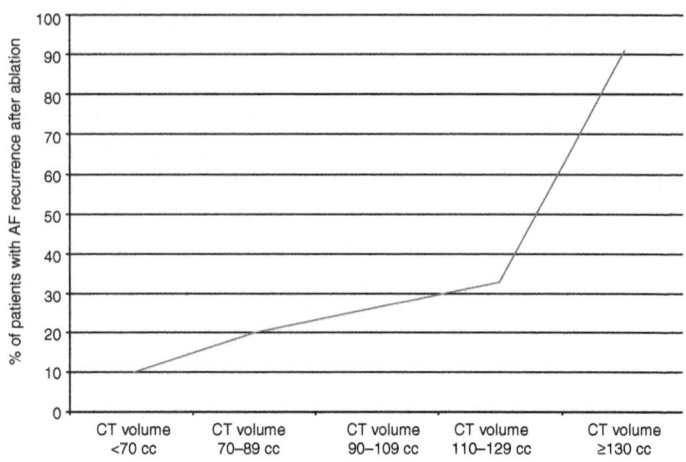

FIGURE 6.1 Failure rate after AF ablation depending on left atrial volume by CT

AF at our institution undergoing AF ablation, left atrial volume measured by CT strongly predicted AF recurrence following ablation. The recurrence rate increased from 10 % in patients with left atrial volumes of less than 70 cc and increased to over 33 % in patients with left atrial volumes between 110 and 129 cc. In patients with a left atrial volume of 130 cc or larger the recurrence rate after ablation was more than 90 % and appeared to function as a threshold for failure [19] (Fig. 6.1).

As shown in the ROC analysis, the frequency of AF recurrence after ablation increases as left atrial volume increases. The recurrence rate increase from 10 % in patients with small atria with volumes <70 cc and increases to over 33 % in patients with left atrial volumes between 110 and 129 cc. A left atrial volume of at least 130 cc as measured by CT appears to function as a threshold. Failure rate in patients with a volume of 130 cc or larger had an AF recurrence rate of more than 90 %.

Complications of AF Ablation and Anatomic Considerations

Catheter ablation of AF is one of the most complex ablation procedures performed by electrophysiologists. It is therefore expected that AF ablation is associated with more extensive and higher complications rates even in experienced centers. The most recent worldwide survey of AF ablation included 45,115 procedures in 32,569 patients. Thirty two deaths occurred resulting in a mortality rate of 0.98 per 1,000 patients. The most common causes of death included tamponade, stroke, atrioesophageal fistula and massive pneumonia [20]. It should be noted that this data was derived from voluntary surveys and quite possibly significantly underestimates the true morbidity and mortality associated with AF ablation.

Complications associated with AF ablation may be related in part to regional differences in left atrial (LA) transmural wall thickness. In an effort to investigate this, we measured LA wall transmural thickness in 34 human heart specimens using calipers in five anatomic areas frequently targeted during AF ablation (anterior wall, septum, mitral isthmus, posterior wall and roof). The roof was the thinnest region measuring significantly less than each other area. The septum was the thickest area [21]. Significant regional differences exist among the different anatomic areas within the left atrium and lower power and temperature should be used in anatomic regions within the left atrium known to have thinner transmural wall thickness.

Approach to the Left Atrium

Transseptal Puncture

Transseptal puncture (TSP) is the conventional approach to accessing the left atrium. TSP can be challenging even for experienced physicians. In our laboratory we rely on several fluoroscopic and intracardiac images when performing TSP. The

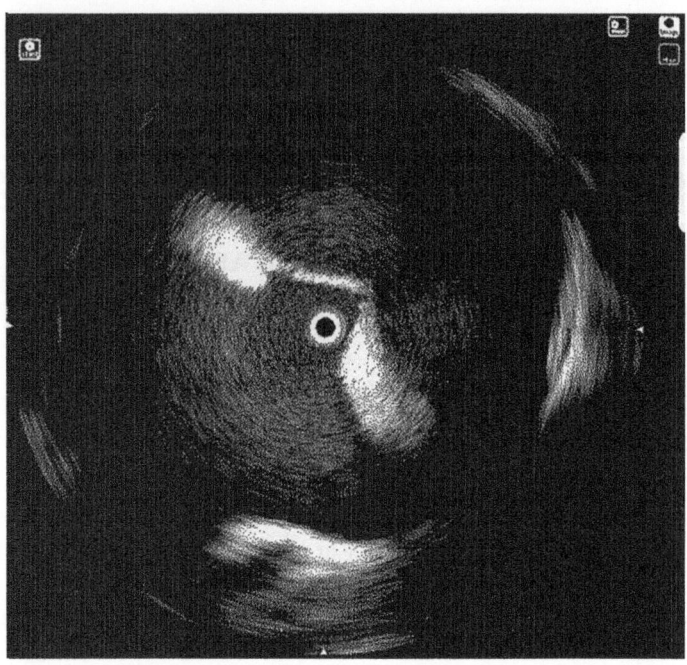

FIGURE 6.2 ICE image showing clear tenting of the fossa ovalis prior to transseptal puncture

intracardiac echo (ICE) catheter is placed in the superior vena cava (SVC) viewed from the anterior posterior (AP) fluoroscopic view. The ICE catheter is then pulled down inferiorly in the AP view until the fossa ovalis is clearly visualized. At this point it is important to view the anatomic relationship of the ICE catheter and the os of the coronary sinus identified by the coronary sinus catheter. Positioning the ICE catheter too inferiorly and thus closer to the coronary sinus os may result in a TSP location that is too low which can allow the trans-septal needle to fall into the right ventricle when applying forward pressure at the time of the puncture. Once a clear image of the fossa ovalis is seen, the transseptal needle is advanced into the introducer of the guide sheath and pulled down from the SVC in the AP view until clear tenting is seen on the ICE image (Fig. 6.2). We prefer to perform the actual puncture in the left anterior oblique

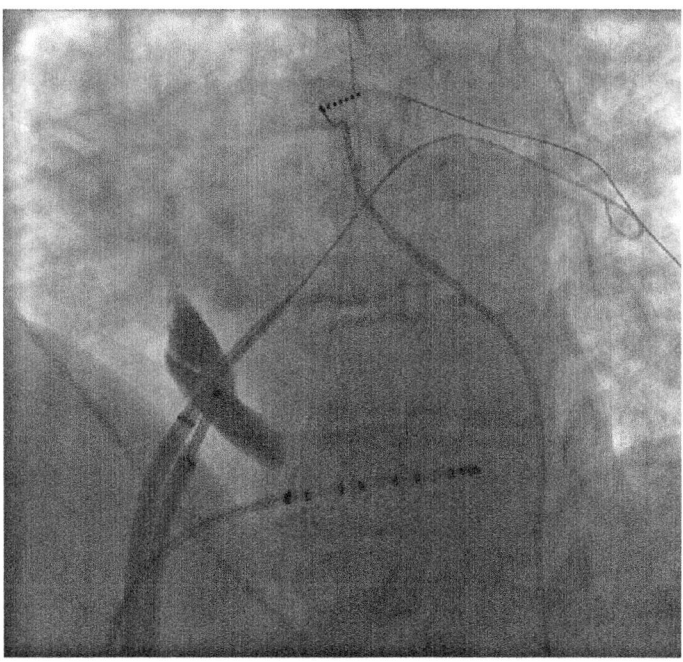

FIGURE 6.3 A guide wire is advanced into the left superior pulmonary vein after the introducer enters the left atrium. This serves as a guide when advancing the sheath to prevent the sheath/introducer combination from forcibly hitting the left atrial free wall

(LAO) fluoroscopic view and the camera is moved from an AP view to 40° LAO at this time. At this point forward pressure is applied to the sheath and introducer until further tenting is seen. The trans-septal needle is then advanced until the fossa ovalis is crossed. It is our preference to use a radiofrequency powered transseptal needle as we have found that this results in high success rates and lower fluoroscopy times. Confirmation of the trans-septal needle location is then assessed by injecting contrast dye with the aid of a manifold into the needle hub. The transseptal needle is then removed from the body leaving the sheath introducer just across the fossa with the tip in the left atrium. A 0.32 guide wire is then advanced through the introducer into the left superior pulmonary vein (Fig. 6.3). It is only after this step that the sheath is advanced into the left atrium by pushing the sheath and introducer at the same time over the guide wire. At times it can take moderate applied pressure to advance the sheath into the left atrium. Advancing the sheath across a guide wire placed in the left superior pulmonary vein prevents the sheath and introducer from forcibly hitting the free wall of the left atrium as it is advanced.

Catheter Manipulation Within the Left Atrium and Pulmonary Veins

Once access to the left atrium has been achieved, we routinely inject contrast into the left and right pulmonary veins (Figs. 6.4 and 6.5). Despite the fact that we utilize three

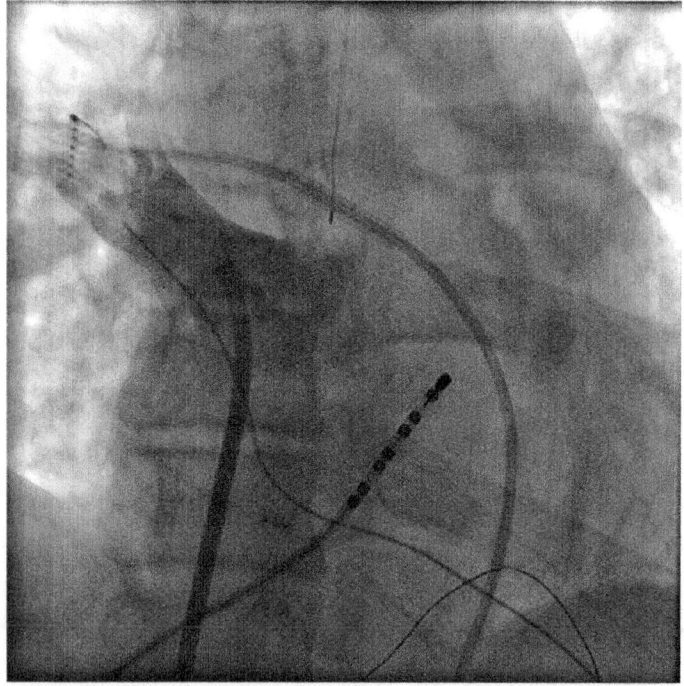

FIGURE 6.4 Contrast injection into the right superior pulmonary vein

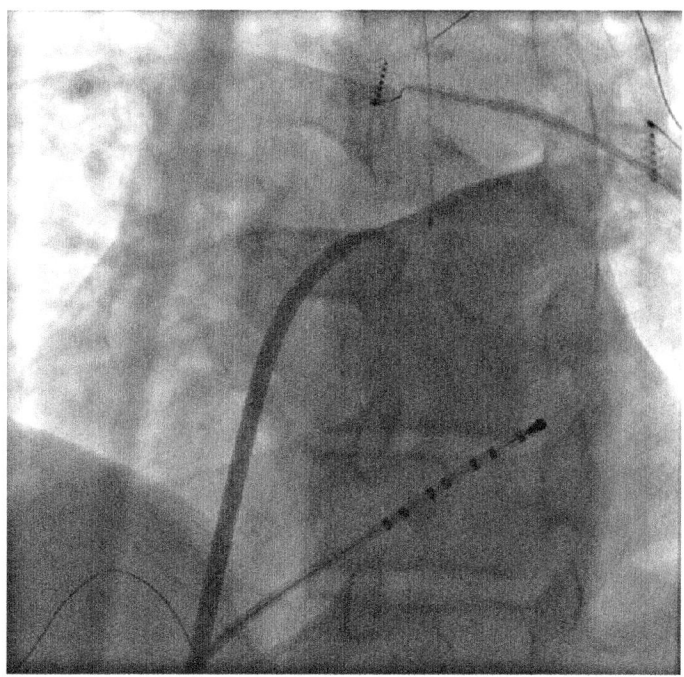

Figure 6.5 Contrast injection into the left superior pulmonary vein. Also seen is the esophageal temperature probe posterior to the vein

dimensional electroanatomical mapping it is still very useful to have a fluoroscopic image of the pulmonary vein ostia and the relationship of the ostia to the cardiac border and spine which varies significantly between individual patients. This serves to increase the safety of the procedure with fluoroscopic confirmation that the ablation catheter is well outside the pulmonary vein ostia.

Catheter manipulation within the left atrium can be broken down into the pulmonary veins and six major anatomic regions: right anterior wall, right inferior wall, left anterior/ridge, left posterior wall, left atrial roof and appendage. If one were to draw an imaginary line down the middle of the left atrium, it is our preference to use AP or shallow RAO fluoroscopic views when manipulating the ablation catheter to the right of that line and LAO for any catheter movement to the left of that line.

The pulmonary vein ostium are posterior structures within the left atrium. As such posterior torque on the catheter and sheath is necessary to access the veins. The left superior pulmonary vein (LSPV) can be entered by directly advancing the ablation catheter from the trans-septal site with clocking the catheter and sheath in a posterior direction. It can be virtually impossible to define the left atrial appendage from the LSPV on two dimensional fluoroscopy. It is therefore imperative that one carefully looks at the local atrial electrogram as the catheter is being advanced into the LSPV. If the catheter is advanced in too much of an anterior direction, the left atrial appendage can be entered inadvertently and this would be associated with a large amplitude atrial electrogram which should immediately be recognized by the operator. This is in contrast to what one would expect when advancing the catheter in to the LSPV which reveals a diminishing electrogram amplitude. The left inferior pulmonary vein can be entered by maintaining the same posterior torque and advancing the catheter slightly in the inferior direction. The real time impedance should also be carefully monitored. A high impedance (over 110 Ω) would suggest that the catheter is too distal within the pulmonary vein and ablation should then be avoided.

The right superior pulmonary vein (RSPV) is easily accessed by pulling the catheter out of the LSPV and clocking the sheath and catheter across the high posterior wall until the catheter falls into the RSPV. After mapping the RSPV the catheter can be rotated in a further clockwise direction until it falls out of the vein onto the high anterior wall of the left atrium. At this point the sheath and the catheter can be pulled down together in an inferior direction to the level of the trans-septal puncture to obtain the remainder of the anteroseptal wall (Fig. 6.6).

The right inferior pulmonary vein (RIPV) and surrounding left atrium can be one of the most difficult anatomic regions of the left atrium to reach. This is especially true with smaller left atriums where there is very little distance between the trans-septal puncture site and the inferior os of

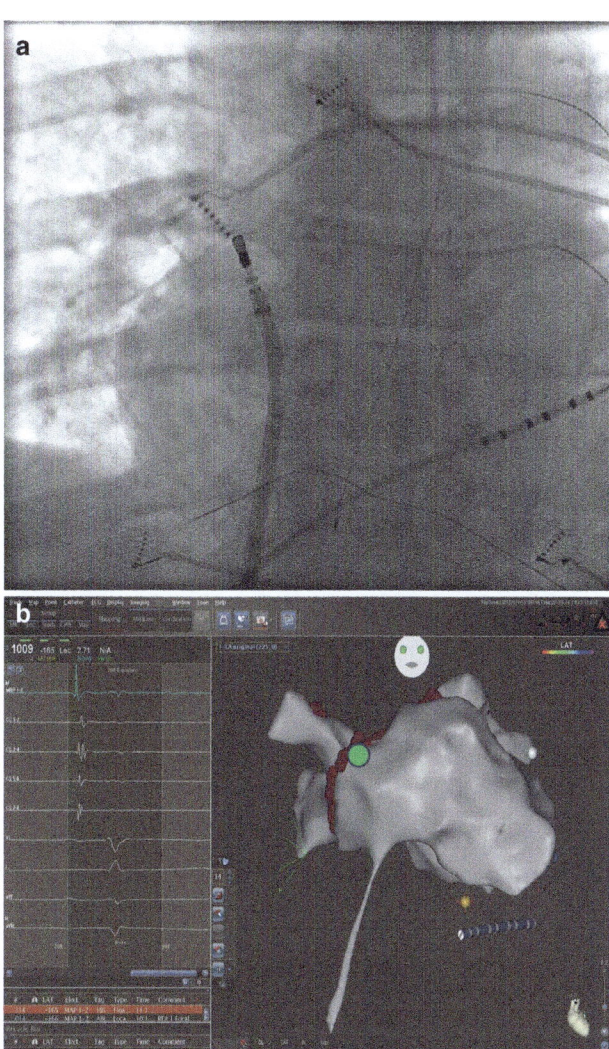

FIGURE 6.6 Approach to anterior wall outside the RSPV. Corresponding fluoroscopic image (**a**) and location (*green circle*) on three dimensional electroanatomical map (**b**). The ablation catheter is rotated in a clockwise direction from inside the RSPV until it falls on the anterior antrum/wall. The ablation catheter and sheath and then pulled sequentially in an inferior direction to map or ablate the remainder of the anterior wall to the level of the trans-septal puncture

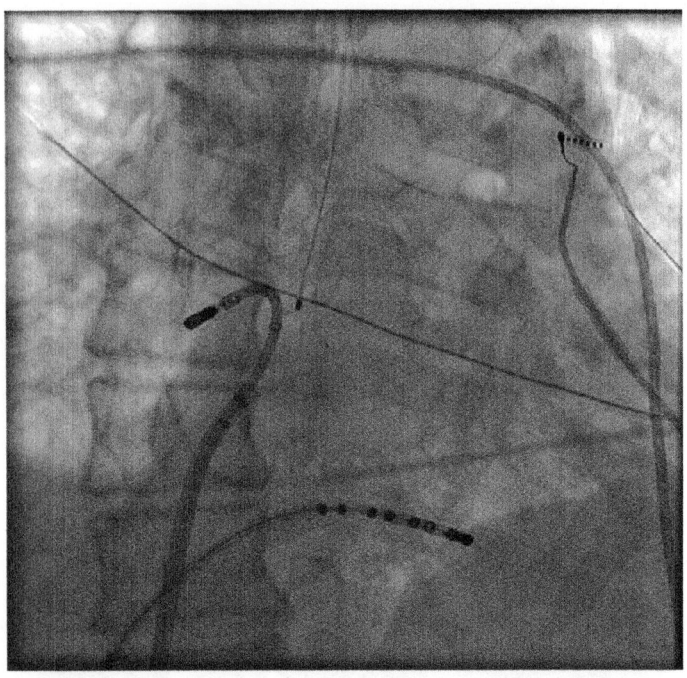

Figure 6.7 Approach to the right posterior wall and right inferior pulmonary vein – Catheter position shown on corresponding AP fluoroscopy and three dimensional electro-anatomical map views. The sheath is directed toward the left and pulled back into the right atrium. The ablation catheter is then positioned in the opposite direction of the sheath and moved in an inferiorly and superiorly to manipulate the entire right posterior wall. Advancing the catheter in this position will access the right inferior pulmonary vein. Also seen is the esophageal temperature probe placed at the level of the distal tip of the ablation catheter

the RIPV. The os of the RIPV is located much more posteriorly than any of the other veins which adds to the challenge of entering this vein and performing ablation around its' entire circumference. When accessing the RIPV, it is our preference to point the sheath toward the LSPV. The catheter is then deflected more than 180° with posterior (counter clockwise torque) until the RIPV is entered (Fig. 6.7). The catheter will not leave the fluoroscopic cardiac silhouette as it does with the other three veins because of the very posterior direction of the RIPV. The right posterior wall and low right anterior wall below the trans-septal puncture site can then be mapped from this configuration by counter clockwise or clockwise catheter rotation respectively.

There are two equally effective methods to both map and ablate along the left atrial roof. The roof of the left atrium is not a flat structure. The roof immediately outside of the LSPV is much more superior than the roof anatomy as it enters the RSPV. This superior to inferior direction of the roof must be taken into account as the catheter is manipulated across the left atrial roof. In an AP fluoroscopic view, the tip of the ablation catheter can be placed in the os of the RSPV with the sheath pointed toward the left. The curvature of the catheter is then relaxed allowing the catheter to fall across the roof from right to left (Fig. 6.8). Alternatively, the catheter can be placed into the os of the LSPV. The catheter and sheath are then clocked together in a sequential fashion across the posterior aspect of the roof until the os of the RSPV is reached. With this method local esophageal temperature must be carefully monitored given the more posterior roof line that is created.

The ridge of the left atrium is located between the anterior os of the LSPV and the left atrial appendage. There is significant anatomic variation to this structure between patients. Higher power settings are often required to achieve bidirectional electrical block along the ridge. The ridge can be ablated from the pulmonary venous or appendage side. It is our preference to ablate along the venous side of the ridge. The ablation catheter is advanced into the LSPV and the sheath is advanced well into the left atrium over the catheter. The catheter is then withdrawn as counterclockwise torque is applied to the sheath. Ablation is performed when both an acceptable electrogram and impedance is obtained. This is one area of the left atrium where more sheath support is required. Without the sheath support, small anterior or posterior movements of the catheter will cause it to fall into the left atrial appendage or LSPV respectively (Fig. 6.9).

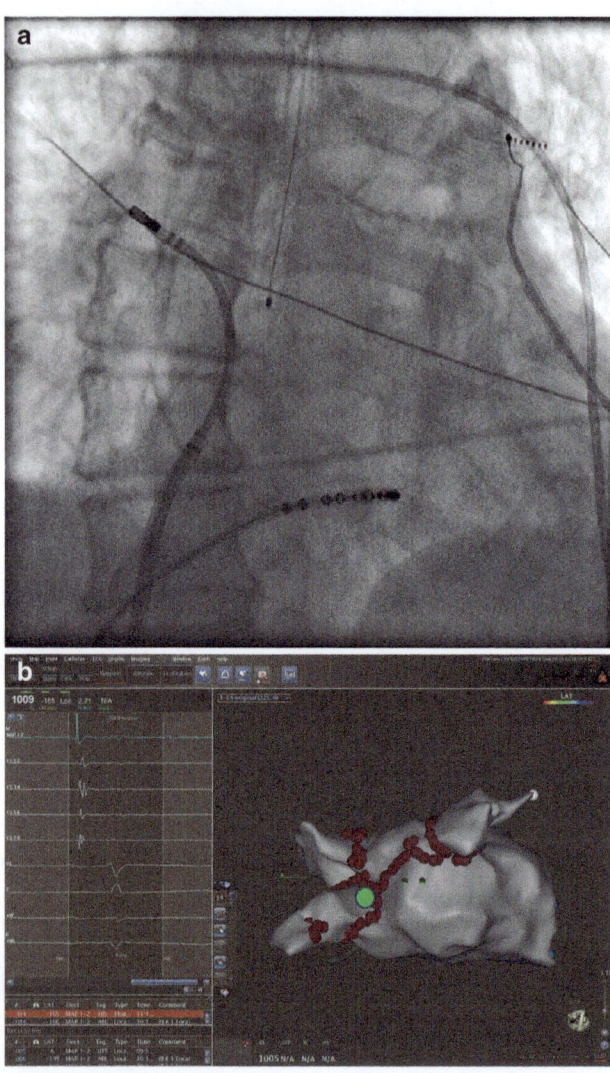

FIGURE 6.8 Corresponding catheter position in AP fluoroscopic (**a**) and three dimensional electro-anatomical map (**b**) (*green circle*) views. To obtain the left atrial roof anatomy the sheath is pointed to the left and the ablation catheter is positioned in the opposite direction with the tip just outside the right superior pulmonary vein. From this position, the catheter curve is slowly released, thus allowing the catheter to sweep the roof and ends at the ostium of the left superior pulmonary vein

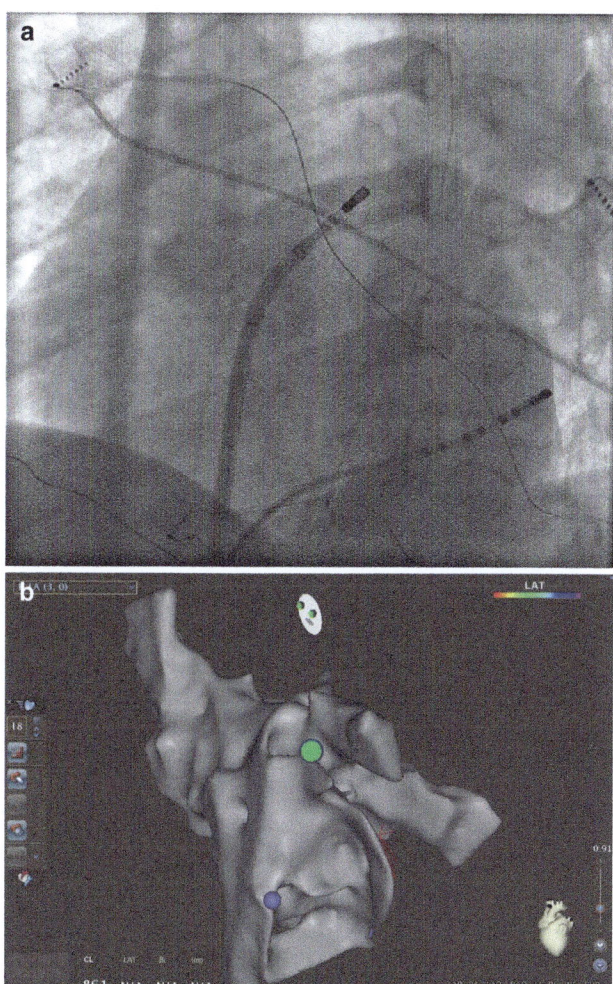

FIGURE 6.9 Catheter manipulation at the left atrial ridge between the LSPV and appendage. Corresponding fluoroscopic (**a**) views and on three dimensional electroanatomical map (**b**) (*green circle*). The ablation catheter is advanced into the LSPV. Counter clockwise anterior torque is then applied to the sheath and catheter as the catheter is pulled back into the sheath until it lands on the ridge. Further counterclockwise rotation will cause the catheter to fall into the appendage

The left atrial appendage is usually easily mapped. It is one of the most anterior structures within the left atrium. Advancing the catheter from the trans-septal site toward the LSPV with substantially more anterior torque will allow the catheter to fall into the appendage. It is important to predominately map the base of the appendage because advancing the catheter too far into the appendage can dramatically increase the risk of perforation is unnecessary for the ablation of AF. In some patients the left atrial appendage can protrude anteriorly over the mitral annulus rather than in the more common anterior superior direction. This anatomic variation should be recognized if no clear left atrial appendage is seen in the usual anatomic location.

Remote Magnetic Navigation-Guided Pulmonary Vein Isolation

Remote magnetic navigation (RMN) catheter ablation has recently been shown to be a feasible and safe technique to achieve PVI with long-term effectiveness [22, 23]. Potential advantages of RMN catheter ablation are catheter contact and stability as well as the potential for reduced risk of complications secondary to the atraumatic design of the RMN ablation catheter. We recently described our own experience with RMN for the ablation of AF in 30 consecutive patients [24]. Seventy seven percent of this small patient cohort had persistent atrial fibrillation with an average left atrial volume of 95.4 ± 33.2 ml. These patients were compared to 61 patients undergoing AF ablation with a standard PVI ablation procedure. The rates of final PVI for the individual pulmonary veins for RMN and standard PVI approaches were similar (86.7 % versus 89.8 % respectively, $p = 0.67$) (Fig. 6.10). However, we did find that anatomic ablation alone with RMN catheter ablation was insufficient to achieve acceptable rates of PVI. In other words, even though RMN catheter ablation may offer improved catheter stability and endocardial contact during radiofrequency application, it is still necessary to utilize an

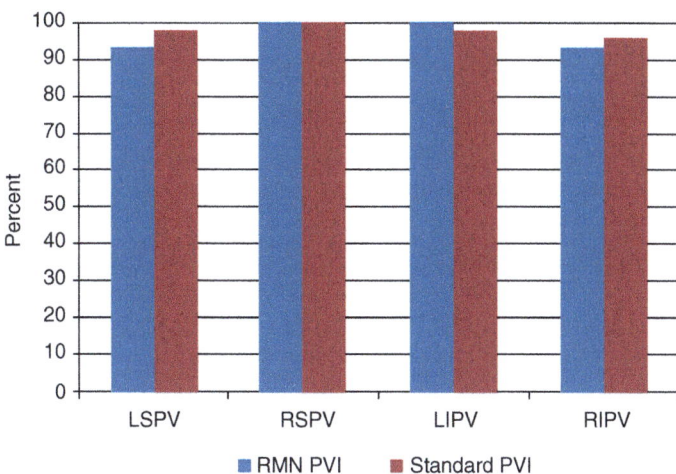

F_IGURE_ 6.10 Final individual pulmonary vein isolation rates for remote magnetic navigation and standard ablation techniques. *LSPV* left superior pulmonary vein, *LIPV* left inferior pulmonary vein, *RSPV* right superior pulmonary vein, *RIPV* right inferior pulmonary vein

electrogram based approach with a circumferential 20 pole catheter (Lasso) within the pulmonary vein ostium to insure high rates of electrical isolation. No significant procedural complications were noted with either the standard or RMN-guided PVI.

Left Atrial Tachycardia Following Left Atrial Ablation for Atrial Fibrillation

As left atrial circumferential ablation has become a more effective and common therapy for atrial fibrillation [12, 25], one of the potential complicating features is the development of LA macroreentrant and focal tachycardias in the post ablation period [26, 27].

Prevalence and Incidence of Left Atrial Tachycardia Following LA Circumferential Ablation

The reported prevalence and incidence of left atrial tachycardia following LA ablation varies between medical centers. Chugh et al. reported that 20 % of patients in one series of 349 patients undergoing LA circumferential ablation had either spontaneous or induced left atrial tachycardia in the electrophysiology lab following the ablation procedure. In these patients, 55 % subsequently developed spontaneous LA tachycardia during follow-up. Overall, 24 % of patient undergoing LA circumferential ablation developed spontaneous left atrial tachycardia during an average follow-up of 394 ± 144 days post ablation. Among the 24 % of patients who developed spontaneous left atrial tachycardia during follow-up, 53 % of these had not had any left atrial tachycardia during the index ablation procedure [26]. Mesas et al. reported a lower incidence of left atrial tachycardia following circumferential left atrial ablation. In their series of 276 patients undergoing left atrial circumferential ablation, 13 patient developed left atrial tachycardia during follow-up for an approximate incidence of 4.7 %. It is not known how many patients in this series developed acute left atrial tachycardia in the electrophysiology laboratory. All of these patients underwent ablation for their left atrial tachycardia at a mean duration of 2.6 ± 1.6 months following the ablation procedure [27].

Left atrial tachycardia will most commonly occur within the first 4 weeks following the ablation procedure. Chugh et al. reported that spontaneous atrial tachycardia occurred at a mean of 44 ± 62 days following ablation with 58 % of these atrial tachycardias occurring within 4 weeks of the procedure [26]. Mesas et al. report a mean time interval between the ablation procedure and occurrence of atrial tachycardia of 2.6 ± 1.6 months [27]. However, one could assume that these patients may have had earlier occurrence of left atrial tachycardia given the fact that all of these patients also underwent ablation for left atrial tachycardia at the same time interval of 2.6 ± 1.6 months post left atrial circumferential ablation.

A significant proportion of patients who develop left atrial tachycardia following LA circumferential ablation will have spontaneous termination of their arrhythmia. This is likely the result of ongoing fibrosis within the left atrium that may lead to elimination of gaps over time that where initially present in the immediate post ablation period. This should be taken into account when making a decision regarding the timing of ablation for left atrial tachycardia. Approximately one-third of atrial tachycardias following LA circumferential ablation will resolve spontaneously within 2–5 months following the ablation procedure. On rare occasion, left atrial tachycardia can take up to 6 months for spontaneous resolution [26]. Thus, an ablation procedure for left atrial tachycardia following ablation for atrial fibrillation should be deferred for 3–4 months to allow for spontaneous resolution.

Treatment of LA Tachycardia Following LA Circumferential Ablation

Treatment of left atrial tachycardia occurring within the first 3 months following LA circumferential ablation should initially include direct current cardioversion. If the patient is on antiarrhythmic drug therapy, a trial off antiarrhythmic drugs can be attempted given the potential proarrhythmic effect of these drugs post ablation. In patients who fail cardioversion and who are not on antiarrhythmic drugs, initiation of amiodarone or a class IC drug may prove effective. For patients who fail both antiarrhythmic therapy and repeat cardioversion, rate control with beta-blockers and calcium channel blockers should be used until either spontaneous resolution occurs or an ablation procedure is performed.

Patients who fail to have spontaneous resolution of LA tachycardia within 4 months following their ablation procedure will require a second ablation procedure to terminate their left atrial tachycardia. Ablation of LA tachycardia following LA circumferential ablation can be very challenging. There are multiple areas of scar within the left atrium following ablation for atrial fibrillation and many potential gap sites exist in the previous ablation lines. It can also be very difficult to capture local myocardium within the left atrium in the post ablation state with the mapping/ablation catheter. This makes the post pacing interval impossible to perform at times and it can be unreliable if very high output is required to obtain local atrial capture. The first step in performing an ablation for left atrial tachycardia should be to create a very detailed activation map of the left atrium with a three dimensional electroanatomic mapping system. This will immediately allow for differentiation between a focal vs. a macroreentrant arrhythmia. Any site that clearly exhibits a very fractionated local electrogram should be tagged as these sites may represent local gaps within previous ablation lines. Perhaps the most helpful maneuver to perform when attempting ablation for left atrial tachycardia is the post pacing interval when local capture is possible. Any site where the post pacing interval is within 20 ms of the tachycardia cycle length is certainly within the reentrant circuit in the case of macroreentrant LA tachycardia. Ablation should be performed between anatomical obstacles when the intervening tissue has a good post pacing interval. Sites with widely split double potentials should also be considered for potential ablation sites as these may represent local gaps. Given the often incessant nature and symptomatology of left atrial tachycardia, aggressive reinduction techniques should be employed after initial termination of left atrial tachycardia in the electrophysiology lab to ensure that the substrate no longer exist for the left atrial tachycardia. Rapid atrial pacing should be performed both without and with the addition of isoproterenol. Despite the challenges of ablation for LA tachycardia, the overall success rate is quite high. Acute success rates of 88 and 93 % were reported by Chugh et al. and Mesas et al. respectively [26, 27].

Origin and Mechanisms of LA Tachycardia Following LA Circumferential Ablation

Given the extensive ablation that is required for LA circumferential ablation, there exist a multitude of potential arrhythmogenic foci for LA tachycardia. The mitral isthmus is a common critical isthmus for left atrial tachycardia following ablation for atrial fibrillation. Chugh et al. found that all the left atrial tachycardias in their series were macroreentrant in origin and that the critical isthmus was localized to the mitral isthmus in 61 % of patients. In the remainder of patients the critical isthmus was localized to the septum (18 %), LA roof (14 %) and coronary sinus (7 %) [26]. Mesas et al. reported a more varied location of the left atrial tachycardias seen in that series of 13 patients undergoing LA tachycardia ablation following LA circumferential ablation. Three patients had a focal origin of their LA tachycardia originating from the septal aspect of the right pulmonary veins in two patients and from the superior segment of the lateral LA in the third patient. The remainder of the patients had macroreentrant arrhythmias. The critical component of the circuit was localized to the mitral isthmus in three patients, the septum (both inferior and superior) in six patients and the lateral-superior wall in one patient [27].

It is important to prove electrical block across ablation lines created for either mitral isthmus or left atrial roof dependent flutter. Mitral isthmus block is best assessed by pacing medial to the ablation line from the left atrial appendage or similar location. When mitral isthmus block is complete, one will see proximal to distal coronary sinus activation when pacing medially from the left atrial appendage (Fig. 6.11). Differential coronary sinus pacing can also be utilized. The timing from distal CS pacing to left atrial

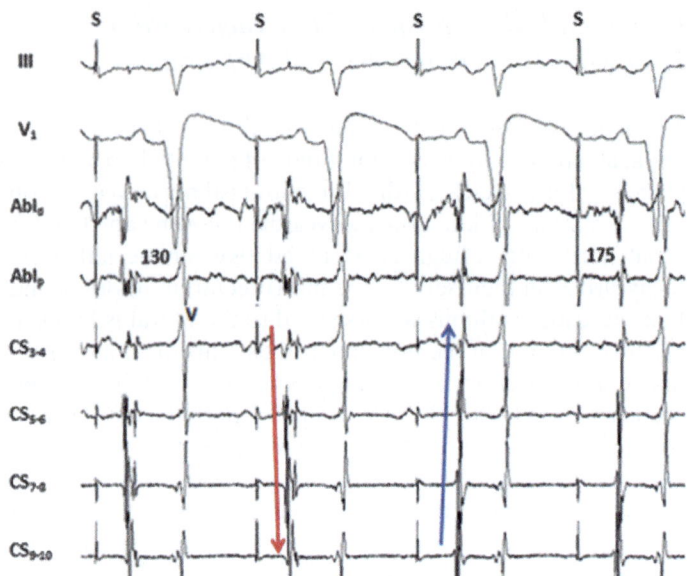

FIGURE 6.11 Mitral isthmus block during ablation on the mitral isthmus and pacing from the left atrial appendage ("S"). "V" = far field ventricular electrogram (Courtesy of Dr. Aman Chugh)

appendage recording will be longer than proximal coronary sinus pacing to the same location when mitral isthmus electrical block is complete.

Electrical block across the left atrial roof can be assessed during normal sinus rhythm without employing pacing maneuvers. Atrial activation normally occurs in a superior to inferior direction as the atrial wave front emerges from the sinus node and then travels across Bachman's bundle to the left atrium. When electrical block across the left atrial roof is complete, the left atrial activation will now occur in a inferior to superior direction. This can be assessed by placing the mapping catheter along the posterior wall of the left atrium in an inferior to superior configuration. When electrical block across the left atrial roof in achieved, the atrial activation will first occur in the distal electrode prior to activating the

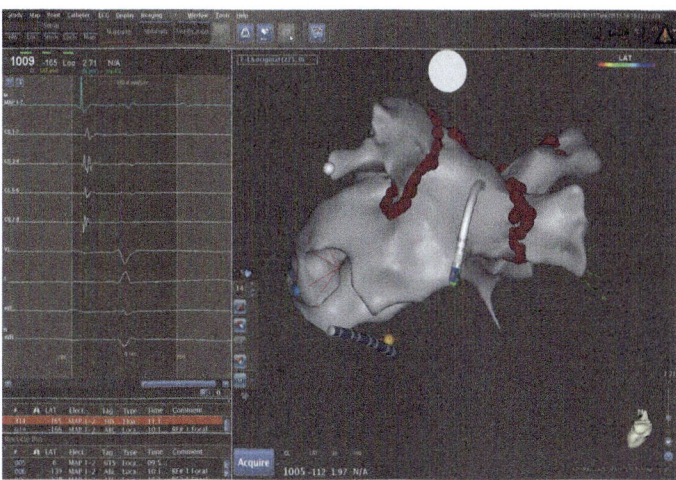

FIGURE 6.12 Roof block. The ablation/mapping catheter is positioned along the posterior wall of the left atrium in an inferior to superior configuration. Distal to proximal atrial activation is seen on the mapping catheter consistent with roof block while in normal sinus rhythm

proximal electrode consistent with a inferior to superior atrial wave front in normal sinus rhythm (Fig. 6.12).

The role of the coronary sinus as a potential origin of LA tachycardia following LA circumferential ablation is always a potential source. The musculature of the coronary sinus has been described as an arrhythmogenic source for both focal and macroreentrant left atrial tachycardias [28, 29]. In a series of 40 patients who underwent mapping and ablation of left atrial tachycardia that developed either during or after LA circumferential ablation, 27 % of these patients were found to have a coronary sinus origin of their tachycardia. The coronary sinus arrhythmia was macroreentrant in 88 % of patients and focal in 12 %. Radiofrequency ablation of the coronary sinus arrhythmia with an 8-mm-tip catheter was acutely successful in 94 % of cases [30]. It is reasonable to rule out the coronary sinus

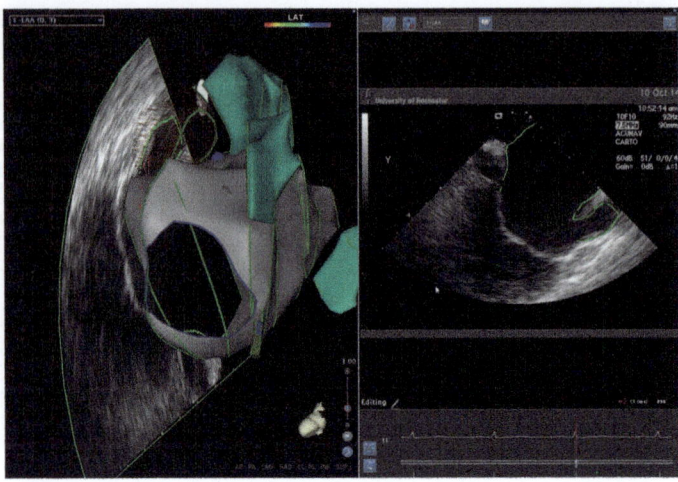

FIGURE 6.13 AF mapping with CartoSound. The *green lines* (contours) in the *right image* create the map in the *left image*. This allows for creation of anatomical geometry with real-time volume of the LA

musculature as a critical component of left atrial tachycardia prior to performing a trans-septal catheterization. If the post pacing interval from the coronary sinus is accurate, ablation can be performed within the coronary sinus to see if the arrhythmia can be successful eliminated without the need for trans-septal catheterization. It is possible to damage the right coronary artery and/or the left circumflex artery when performing ablation within the coronary sinus. However, Chugh et al. reported no coronary artery complications when ablating within the coronary sinus often at power settings of ≥45 W with a non-irrigated tip ablation catheter [30]. Ablation within the coronary sinus should not be attempted if the local impedance is very high as this will likely lead to more thrombotic complications (Figs. 6.13 and 6.14).

LA tachycardia is a relatively common complication following left atrial circumferential ablation for atrial fibrillation. It can be a challenging arrhythmia to treat both medically and with catheter ablation. Careful activation mapping

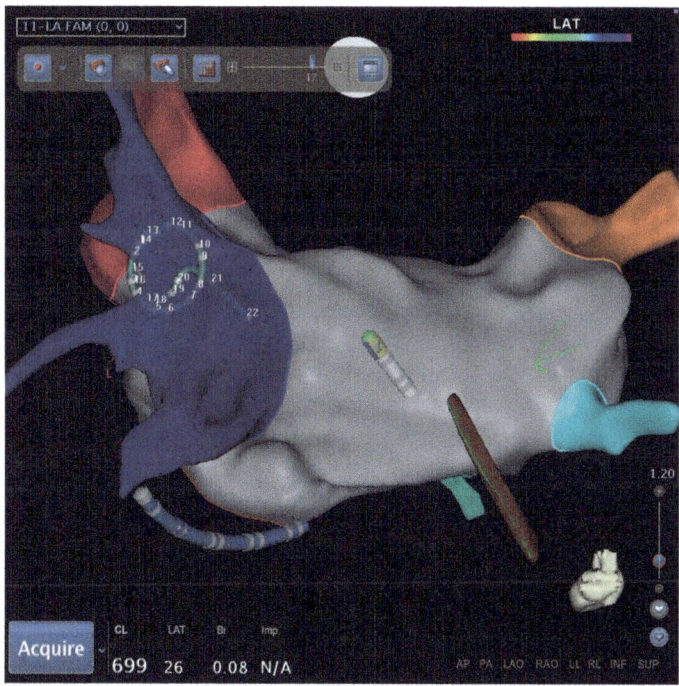

FIGURE 6.14 Combination of mapping strategies with Carto 3 system. This highly detailed map began with CartoSound, prior to crossing septum. Afterwards, the Sound map was used to guide the collection of anatomy with the circular catheter (LA body), and then the mapping catheter. The brown structure is the esophagus, located and mapped with ultrasound, providing a guide to this sensitive structure during ablation on the posterior wall. Notice complex left vein anatomy, and very low, posterior RSPV, which may have been missed without additional imaging technology (Map courtesy of Dr. Steve Zador, Buffalo General Hospital)

and performing post pacing intervals when possible can greatly increase the success when performing ablation. The potential role of the coronary sinus as an arrhythmogenic substrate should always be considered. Finally, ablation for

LA tachycardia should not be performed for several months after the index AF ablation procedure.

Mapping Considerations for AF Ablation

For mapping LA tachycardias, see mapping sections in Chap. 3 on SVT and Chap. 5 on atrial flutter.

While electroanatomic mapping for AF continues to be explored and researched (CFAE, rotor mapping), for the most part AF current remains an anatomical procedure, with focus on isolation of the pulmonary veins. A detailed LA reconstruction is therefore crucial for AF ablation. There is a wide variety of differences in PV anatomy. The simplest form of 3D anatomical mapping for AF is to use the ablation catheter to collect the LA anatomy, with no other assistance. The advantage if this is the ability to get a good feel for the atrium with the ablation catheter while mapping. Disadvantages include the possibility of missing veins and the extra time required to gather a detailed map with a 4-pole catheter. The map can be gathered more rapidly by using multipolar circular catheters designed for verifying PV isolation.

Additional help for mapping comes from technologies that utilize various imaging modalities to see the LA anatomy in real time through phased-array ultrasound imaging or ahead of time through CT or MRI imaging. Regarding the latter, currently available 3D mapping systems can import CT or MRI studies and then segment out the LA in 3 dimensions. This allows for the LA and PVs to be seen ahead of time, taking away the guesswork of PV anatomy. Regarding the former, phased array intracardiac echo (ICE) can be used both for the transseptal puncture and to visualize the LA, LAA, and PVs. The Carto system integrates phased array ICE into its system, allowing the 3D map to be built with the ultrasound images before crossing the septum. The advantage here is limiting the time in the LA by doing a significant amount of 3D mapping before crossing the septum. CartoSound technology also allows for confirmation of catheter-tissue contact by showing the tip of the sensor-based catheter on the integrated ICE image. (See Media)

Anticoagulation Strategies for Ablation of Atrial Fibrillation

The procedural complications associated with AF ablation have decreased in recent years due to improved techniques and operator experience. However, both bleeding and thromboembolic complications continue to be a major source of morbidity for patients undergoing AF ablation. The optimal strategy for periprocedural anticoagulation remains a subject of debate amongst electrophysiologist. There is general agreement; however, that whatever strategy is chosen by the operator should attempt to maximize the appropriate balance between bleeding and thrombosis.

It is now accepted that uninterrupted periprocedural warfarin therapy (with a target international ratio between 2 and 3) is superior to other interrupted anticoagulation strategies [31–35]. A recent meta-analysis included a total of 27,402 patients undergoing AF ablation with either continuous warfarin therapy or discontinuation of warfarin with periprocedural bridging with heparin. In this analysis there were 6,400 patients undergoing ablation with continuous warfarin therapy. Continuous warfarin therapy was associated with a major decrease in thromboembolic complications and minor bleeding complications as compared to discontinuing warfarin in the periprocedural period. The primary analysis did not show a significant difference in the rates of major bleeding between the two strategies. Furthermore, major bleeding complications due to pericardial tamponade were not increased with the use of continuous warfarin therapy as long as monitoring was performed with intracardiac echo [32].

Over the last few years, more patients with atrial fibrillation have been anticoagulated with direct thrombin or factor Xa inhibitors. This has complicated the periprocedural anticoagulation management strategy when these patients are referred for AF ablation. Recent studies evaluating the safety and efficacy of dabigatran as a periprocedural anticoagulant have yielded mixed results [36–40]. Lakkireddy et al. recently reported observational data using dabigatran in the periprocedural AF ablation period. In this particular study dabigatran was held on the morning of the day of the ablation procedure. Dabigatran was associated with an increased risk of bleeding and composite of bleeding or embolic complications compared with continuous uninterrupted warfarin. There was trend toward older age and long standing persistent AF in the dabigatran patient cohort that may in part explain some of the differences in complication rates [36]. Winkle et al. found contrasting results when testing the safety of dabigatran in the post AF ablation period in a retrospective study. In this particular study dabigatran was stopped at a variable time interval pre-ablation. There was no difference in the thromboembolic or hemorrhagic complication rates between warfarin and dabigatran [41]. More recently, Maddox et al. published a retrospective study assessing the efficacy of uninterrupted dabigatran as an alternative strategy to continuous warfarin therapy. This study included a total of 463 patients (212 in the dabigatran and 251 in the warfarin group respectively) which is the largest series of patients using uninterrupted dabigatran as a periprocedural anticoagulant published to date. There were no significant differences in the risk of bleeding or thromboembolic complications between the two strategies [42].

Rivaroxaban, a direct factor Xa inhibitor, has recently been evaluated in a multicenter, observational, prospective study of a registry of patients undergoing AF ablation. Patients taking uninterrupted periprocedural rivaroxaban were matched by age, sex and type of AF with an equal number of patients prescribed continuous warfarin therapy who underwent ablation during the same time period. A total of 642 patients were included in the study. There were no differences in major or minor bleeding or embolic complications between the rivaroxaban and warfarin groups in the first 30 days after ablation. The conclusion of this study was that uninterrupted rivaroxaban was as safe and efficacious in patients undergoing AF ablation as uninterrupted warfarin therapy [43]. A randomized controlled trial comparing uninterrupted warfarin with uninterrupted rivaroxaban therapy for AF ablation (VENTURE-AF) is currently enrolling patients and should help to further clarify the role of rivaroxaban as a periprocedural anticoagulant.

Direct thrombin inhibitors and factor Xa inhibitors do not have a readily available antidote at this time. This leads to valid concerns over managing life threatening bleeding complications during AF ablation with concomitant use of these newer anticoagulants. Prothrombin complex concentrate can reverse some of the anticoagulant effects of rivaroxaban [44] but this has not been tested in a clinical setting during life threatening hemorrhage.

An ideal periprocedural anticoagulation strategy for AF ablation has not been clearly defined at this point. The initial results with factor Xa inhibitors are encouraging but further randomized clinical controlled studies evaluating the safety and efficacy of the newer anticoagulants during AF ablation are needed before firm conclusions can be made.

References

1. Feinberg WM, Cornell ES, Nightingale SD, Pearce LA, Tracy RP, Hart RG, Bovill EG. Relationship between prothrombin activation fragment F1.2 and international normalized ratio in patients with atrial fibrillation. Stroke prevention in atrial fibrillation investigators. Stroke. 1997;28:1101–6.
2. Go AS, Hylek EM, Phillips KA, Chang Y, Henault LE, Selby JV, Singer DE. Prevalence of diagnosed atrial fibrillation in adults: national implications for rhythm management and stroke prevention: the anticoagulation and risk factors in atrial fibrillation (ATRIA) study. JAMA. 2001;285:2370–5.
3. Feinberg WM, Blackshear JL, Laupacis A, Kronmal R, Hart RG. Prevalence, age distribution, and gender of patients with atrial fibrillation. Analysis and implications. Arch Intern Med. 1995;155:469–73.
4. Friberg J, Buch P, Scharling H, Gadsbphioll N, Jensen GB. Rising rates of hospital admissions for atrial fibrillation. Epidemiology. 2003;14:666–72.
5. Wattigney WA, Mensah GA, Croft JB. Increasing trends in hospitalization for atrial fibrillation in the United States, 1985 through 1999: implications for primary prevention. Circulation. 2003;108:711–6.
6. Stewart S, MacIntyre K, MacLeod MM, Bailey AE, Capewell S, McMurray JJ. Trends in hospital activity, morbidity and case

fatality related to atrial fibrillation in Scotland, 1986–1996. Eur Heart J. 2001;22:693–701.

7. Dorian P, Jung W, Newman D, Paquette M, Wood K, Ayers GM, Camm J, et al. The impairment of health-related quality of life in patients with intermittent atrial fibrillation: implications for the assessment of investigational therapy. J Am Coll Cardiol. 2000;36:1303–9.

8. Wang TJ, Larson MG, Levy D, Vasan RS, Leip EP, Wolf PA, D'Agostino RB, et al. Temporal relations of atrial fibrillation and congestive heart failure and their joint influence on mortality: the Framingham Heart Study. Circulation. 2003;107: 2920–5.

9. Wolf PA, Abbott RD, Kannel WB. Atrial fibrillation as an independent risk factor for stroke: the Framingham Study. Stroke. 1991;22:983–8.

10. Benjamin EJ, Wolf PA, D'Agostino RB, Silbershatz H, Kannel WB, Levy D. Impact of atrial fibrillation on the risk of death: the Framingham Heart Study. Circulation. 1998;98:946–52.

11. Wyse DG, Waldo AL, DiMarco JP, Domanski MJ, Rosenberg Y, Schron EB, Kellen JC, et al. A comparison of rate control and rhythm control in patients with atrial fibrillation. N Engl J Med. 2002;347:1825–33.

12. Pappone C, Oreto G, Rosanio S, Vicedomini G, Tocchi M, Gugliotta F, Salvati A, et al. Atrial electroanatomic remodeling after circumferential radiofrequency pulmonary vein ablation: efficacy of an anatomic approach in a large cohort of patients with atrial fibrillation. Circulation. 2001;104:2539–44.

13. Oral H, Pappone C, Chugh A, Good E, Bogun F, Pelosi Jr F, Bates ER, et al. Circumferential pulmonary-vein ablation for chronic atrial fibrillation. N Engl J Med. 2006;354:934–41.

14. 2011 ACCF/AHA/HRS focused updates. Circulation. 2011;123:e269–367.

15. Oral H, Chugh A, Oraydin M, et al. Risk of thromboembolic events after percutaneous left atrial radiofrequency ablation of atrial fibrillation. Circulation. 2006;114(8):759–65.

16. Themistoclakis S, Corrado A, Marchlinski FE, et al. The risk of thromboembolism and need for oral anticoagulation after successful atrial fibrillation ablation. J Am Coll Cardiol. 2010;55(8):735–43.

17. Hussein AA, Saliba WI, Martin DO, et al. Natural history and long-term outcomes of ablated atrial fibrillation. Circ Arrhythm Electrophysiol. 2011;4(3):271–8.

18. 2012 HRS/EHRA/ECAS Expert Consensus Statement on catheter and surgical ablation of atrial fibrillation: recommendations for patient selection, procedural techniques, patient management and follow-up, definitions, endpoints, and research trial design. Europace. Heart Rhythm, 2012;9:4.

19. Parikh S, Jons C, Mcnitt S, et al. Predictive capability of left atrial size measured by CT, TEE and TTE for recurrence of atrial fibrillation following radiofrequency catheter ablation. PACE. 2010;33:532–40.

20. Cappato R, Calkins H, Chen SA, et al. Prevalence and causes of fatal outcome in catheter ablation of atrial fibrillation. J Am Coll Cardiol. 2009;53:1798–803.

21. Hall B, Jeevanantham V, Simon R, et al. Variation in left atrial transmural wall thickness at sites commonly targeted for ablation of atrial fibrillation. J Interv Card Electrophysiol. 2006; 17:127–32.

22. Bauernfeind T, Akca F, Schwagten B, et al. The magnetic navigation system allows safety and high efficacy for ablation of arrhythmias. Europace. 2011;13:1015–21.

23. Choi MS, Oh YS, Jang SW, et al. Comparison of magnetic navigation system and conventional method in catheter ablation of atrial fibrillation: is magnetic navigation system more effective and safer than conventional method? Korean Circ J. 2011;41:248–52.

24. Brenyo A, Rao M, Baibav B, et al. Remote magnetic navigation-guided pulmonary vein isolation: a single center experience. J Innovations Card Rhythm Manag. 2013;4:1248–53.

25. Oral H, Scharf C, Chugh A, Hall B, Cheung P, Good E, Veerareddy S, Pelosi Jr F, Morady F. Catheter ablation for paroxysmal atrial fibrillation: segmental pulmonary vein ostial ablation versus left atrial ablation. Circulation. 2003;108:2355–60.

26. Chugh A, Oral H, Lemola K, Hall B, Cheung P, Good E, Tamirisa K, Han J, Bogun F, Plosi Jr F, Morady F. Prevalence, mechanisms, and clinical significance of macroreentrant atrial tachycardia during and following left atrial ablation for atrial fibrillation. Heart Rhythm. 2005;2:464–73.

27. Mesas C, Pappone C, Lang C, Gugliotta F, Tomita T, Vicedomini G, Sala S, Paglino G, Gulletta S, Ferro A, Santinelli V. Left atrial tachycardia after circumferential pulmonary vein ablation for atrial fibrillation. J Am Coll Cardiol. 2004;44:1071–9.

28. Volkmer M, Antz M, Hebe J, Kuck KH. Focal atrial tachycardia originating from the musculature of the coronary sinus. J Cardiovasc Electrophysiol. 2002;13:68–71.

29. Olgin JE, Jayachandran JV, Engelstein E, Groh W, Zipes DP. Atiral macroreentry involving the myocardium of the coronary sinus: a unique mechanism for atypical flutter. J Cardiovasc Electrophysiol. 1998;9:1094–9.

30. Chugh A, Oral H, Good E, Han J, Tamirisa K, Lemola K, Elmouchi D, Tschopp D, Reich S, Igic P, Bogun F, Pelosi Jr F, Morady F. Catheter ablation of atypical atrial flutter and atrial tachycardia within the coronary sinus after left atrial ablation for atrial fibrillation. J Am Coll Cardiol. 2005;46:83–91.

31. Di Biase L, Burkhardt JD, Mohanty P, et al. Periprocedural stroke and management of major bleeding complications in patients undergoing catheter ablation of atrial fibrillation: the impact of periprocedural therapeutic international normalized ratio. Circulation. 2010;121:2550–6.

32. Santangeli P, Di Biase L, Horton R, et al. Ablation of atrial fibrillation under therapeutic warfarin reduces periprocedural complications: evidence from a meta-analysis. Circ Arrhythm Electrophysiol. 2012;5:302–11.

33. Hussein AA, Martin DO, Saliba W, et al. Radiofrequency ablation of atrial fibrillation under therapeutic international normalized ratio: a safe and efficacious periprocedural anticoagulation strategy. Heart Rhythm. 2009;6:1425–9.

34. Hakalahti A, Uusimaa P, Ylitako K, Raatikainen MJ. Catheter ablation of atrial fibrillation in patients with therapeutic oral anticoagulation treatment. Europace. 2011;13:640–5.

35. Wazni OM, Beheiry S, Fahmy T, et al. Atrial fibrillation ablation in patients with therapeutic international normalized ratio: comparison of strategies of anticoagulation management in the periprocedural period. Circulation. 2007;116:2531–4.

36. Lakkireddy D, Reddy YM, Di Biase L, et al. Feasibility and safety of dabigatran versus warfarin for periprocedural anticoagulation in patients undergoing radiofrequency ablation for atrial fibrillation: results from a multicenter prospective registry. J Am Coll Cardiol. 2012;59:1168–74.

37. Kaseno K, Naito S, Nakamura K, et al. Efficacy and safety of periprocedural dabigatran in patients undergoing catheter ablation of atrial fibrillation. Circ J. 2012;76:2337–42.

38. Kim JS, She F, Jongnarangsin K, et al. Dabigatran vs warfarin for radiofrequency catheter ablation of atrial fibrillation. Heart Rhythm. 2013;10:483–9.

39. Bassiouny M, Saliba W, Rickard J, et al. Use of dabigatran for periprocedural anticoagulation in patients undergoing catheter

ablation for atrial fibrillation. Circ Arrhythm Electrophysiol. 2013;6:460–6.

40. Yamaji H, Murakami T, Hina K, Kusachi S. Usefulness of dabigatran etexilate as periprocedural anticoagulation therapy for atrial fibrillation ablation. Clin Drug Investig. 2013;33:409–18.

41. Winkle RA, Mead RH, Engel G, Kong MH, et al. The use of dabigatran immediately after atrial fibrillation ablation. J Cardiovasc Electrophysiol. 2012;23:264–8.

42. Maddox W, Kay GN, Yamada T, et al. Dabigatran versus warfarin therapy for uninterrupted oral anticoagulation during atrial fibrillation ablation. J Cardiovasc Electrophysiol. 2013; 24:861–5.

43. Lakkireddy D, Reddy TM, Di Biase L, et al. Feasibility and safety of uninterrupted rivaroxaban for periprocedural anticoagulation in patients undergoing radiofrequency ablation of atrial fibrillation. J Am Coll Cardiol. 2014;63:982–8.

44. Eerenberg ES, Kamphuisen PW, Sijpkens MK, et al. Reversal of rivaroxaban and dabigatran by prothrombin complex concentrate: a randomized placebo-controlled crossover study in healthy subjects. Circulation. 2011;124:1573–9.

Chapter 7
Ventricular Tachyarrhythmias

Andrew Brenyo, Travis Prinzi, and David T. Huang

Ventricular tachyarrhythmias often are associated with different symptoms and variable prognoses, and therapy needs to be tailored accordingly. A clear understanding of the underlying substrate and how these ventricular tachyarrhythmias develop is critical in the proper treatment of the patients with these conditions.

How Do Arrhythmias Start?

Electrical impulse normally travels through the heart chambers in a very organized and uniform manner. However, disturbances in how electrical signals are initiated or how they propagate through the cardiac chamber can lead to the onset of arrhythmias. In general, there are three mechanisms of how arrhythmias start. A common arrhythmogenesis is impulse

A. Brenyo, MD
Arrhythmia Consultants, Greenville, SC, USA

T. Prinzi, MD • D.T. Huang, MD (✉)
Department of Cardiology, University of Rochester
Medical Center, Rochester, NY, USA
e-mail: David_Huang@URMC.Rochester.edu

D.T. Huang, T. Prinzi (eds.), *Clinical Cardiac Electrophysiology in Clinical Practice*, In Clinical Practice, DOI 10.1007/978-1-4471-5433-4_7,
© Springer-Verlag London 2015

reentry. Tissues may intrinsically exhibit multiple pathways (as in dual atrioventricular nodal physiology, see "Chap. 3 SVT") or develop multiple pathways in the healing process (as in scars post myocardial infarction) through which the electrical signal may travel. If these paths are associated with different conduction velocities and correspondingly different refractory periods, the electrical signals can circle around in an "endless loop" through these circuit paths. Conditions suitable for reentry require the slower conducting pathway to have a shorter refractory period and the faster conducting pathway to have a longer refractory period. Most VTs, though certainly not all, related to post myocardial infarction substrate or cardiomyopathy are due to impulse reentry. Monomorphic VT is often due to stable and fixed circuits of reentry whereas polymorphic VT can be due to unstable and meandering or even multiple circuits of reentry. Another mechanism for arrhythmia onset is due to triggered activity. Increased intracellular calcium concentration due to heightened adrenergic stimulation (such as exercise) initiates a cascade of reaction through activation of stimulatory G proteins, resulting in enhanced calcium entry through the cellular calcium channels and calcium induced calcium release in the sarcoplasmic reticulum. This increase in the intracellular calcium may then activate the sodium calcium exchanger leading to abnormal sodium entry into the cell which may trigger depolarization of the heart cell, resulting in premature beats or even tachycardia [1]. Forms of normal heart idiopathic ventricular tachycardia associated with exercise, such as one originating right ventricular outflow tract, are often resulting from triggered activity. A third mechanism for arrhythmogenesis is enhanced automaticity, where cardiac muscle tissue develops spontaneous electrical activity through abnormal depolarization during phase 4 of the action potential. These arrhythmias are usually referred as "automatic" tachycardia. Some examples of these include variants of tachycardia related to diseased tissue where the baseline membrane potential may be unstable. Typically, sources of tachycardia that are focal are due to either triggered activity or enhanced automaticity.

The management of ventricular arrhythmias is thus complex and quite variable, with this variance discussed in the following segments. Our initial focus will be scar mediated VT (VT with an abnormal left ventricular ejection fraction [LVEF]) followed by idiopathic PVC's and less frequent forms of idiopathic ventricular tachycardia (VT with a normal LVEF).

Electrocardiographic Evaluation of Ventricular Arrhythmias

The first and most important diagnostic tool remains the 12 lead electrocardiogram during a wide QRS complex tachycardia. Often the type of cardiomyopathy, location of scarring, and VT exit can be estimated from the appearance of the tachycardia. Multiple algorithms have been developed and studied for the electrocardiographic diagnosis of VT including the Brugada criteria [2] and various individual lead (Lead II, AVR) [3, 4] analysis techniques, all with good specificity and sensitivity for the identification of VT in distinction from supraventricular tachyarrhythmias (SVT) with aberrancy. All these algorithms take advantage of the initial forces of activation to distinguish VT from SVT. Tachycardia of ventricular origin depolarizes the myocardial muscles by cell-to-cell contact and thus will have slower forces of activation represented by delayed or fragmented portions early in the QRS signals. On the other hand, during SVT, even with aberrancy, the heart muscles are activated via engaging the specialized conduction tissues and are generally associated with a more smooth and rapid initial QRS signals. Of note, all of these algorithms are qualified and should be used with caution in patients with manifest preexcitation (i.e., Wolff-Parkinson-White syndrome) or on antiarrhythmic medical therapy. Updated morphology criteria developed in recent years have resulted in more elegant and simplified algorithm to decipher whether a wide complex tachycardia may be VT or SVT with aberrancy. Inspecting the morphology of the initial QRS signals in lead aVR can be used to suggest ventricular origin of a wide complex tachycardia. As illustrated in

Fig. 7.1, QRS with slow or notched initial forces as well as those with unusual axis all suggest a diagnosis of VT rather than SVT. Similarly, if the duration of the QRS signal from the beginning of the onset to the peak of the R wave in lead II measures to be greater or equal to 50 ms, then VT can be diagnosed with better than 95 % confidence (Figs. 7.1, 7.2, and 7.3).

Once diagnosis is made that the arrhythmia is VT, the next step is to determine the activation vector of the ventricle. As a simplistic starting point, the bundle branch block appearance of the QRS complex indicates the culprit chamber where the VT is originating from. A left bundle branch block appearance indicates an RV or septal LV VT while a right bundle branch appearance indicates an LV VT origin. Taking this approach a step further, using the right sided leads (V1, AVR), inferior leads (II/III/AVF), lateral leads (1/AVL) and apical leads (V5/V6) one can identify where the VT is coming from

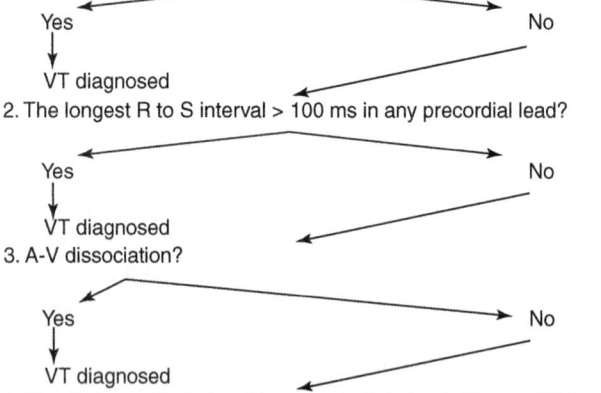

FIGURE 7.1 Algorithm to determine VT vs. SVT by Brugada et al. [2] (Used with permission)

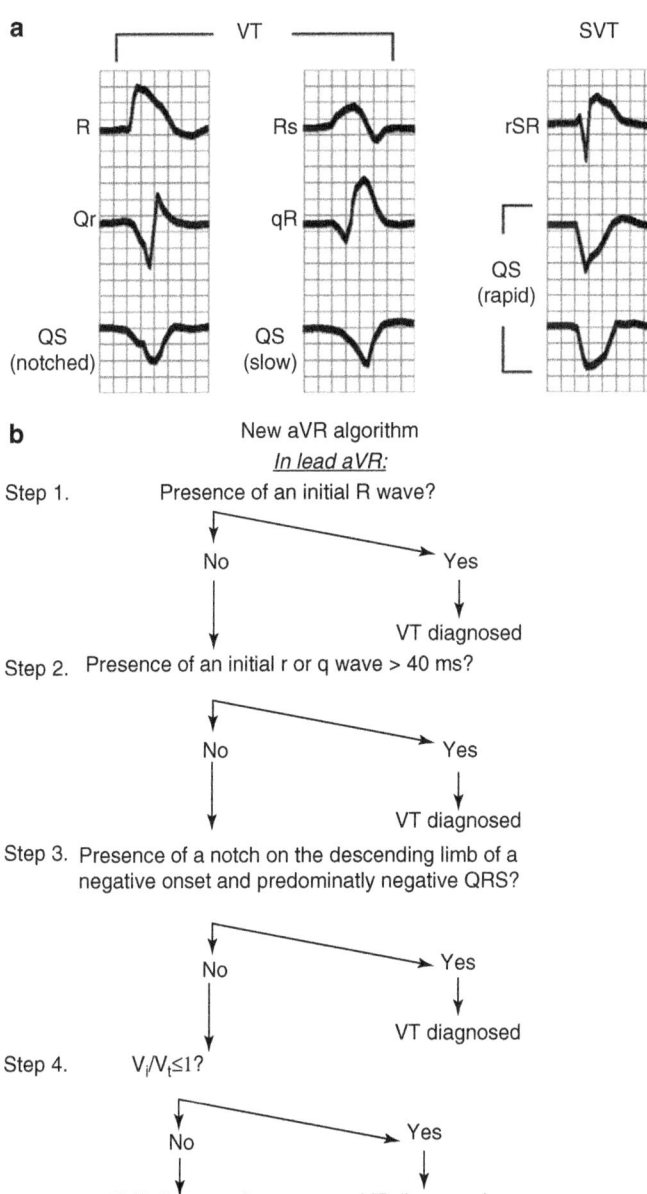

FIGURE 7.2 Algorithm to determine VT vs SVT with aberrancy by criteria developed in aVR. (**a**) By aVR QRS morphologies. (**b**) Algorithm decision ladder (Used with permission)

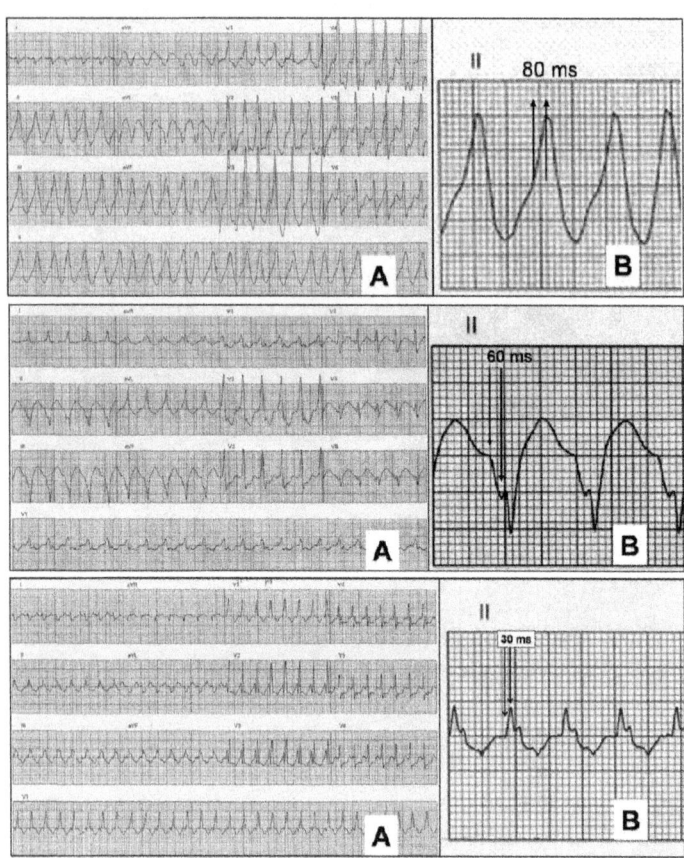

FIGURE 7.3 Algorithm to determine VT vs. SVT by measuring the duration of onset of QRS to the peak of R wave lead II. Signals measuring ≥50 ms (*top two panels*) suggest VT whereas <50 ms suggest SVT with aberrancy [4] (Used with permission)

(negative QS vector) and going towards (positive RS vector). Generally, biphasic QRS vectors mean that the origin is somewhere in the middle of that individual vector, i.e. a biphasic QRS vector in 1 and V1 likely indicate that the origin/exit site of the VT is in the septum and not on the right (RV, Q wave in V1) or left (posterior LV, Q wave in 1). This approach is primarily useful in reentrant VT's and idiopathic PVC's.

A close examination of the resting 12 lead ECG can also provide significant clues as to the underlying process and likely culprit areas of myocardial scarring. The presence of Q waves in the distribution of a coronary artery should indicate the presence of scarring that will often play a critical role in sustaining VT. Fragmentation (extra notching) of the surface QRS complex in a similar distribution to a major coronary vessel and Q waves often can provide a more sensitive indicator of myocardial scarring and may indicate the presence of epicardial scarring in that region.

For idiopathic VT's such as RVOT and LVOT VT, the appearance should be consistent with an outflow origin (inferior axis, i.e., positive in the inferior leads II/III/AVF) with an earlier precordial transition (V3 or less) indicating an LV origin and a later transition (V3 or later) indicating an RV origin. Transition at V3 could represent either LV or RV origin. Idiopathic VT utilizing the conduction system (bundle branch and fasicular reentry VT's) are quite uncommon but do have characteristic features that should set them aside from VT associated with structural heart disease. The VT is generally slower with a typical bundle branch or fasicular block appearance during tachycardia that is usually very similar to the appearance of the baseline QRS complex at rest Figure 7.12. Bundle branch and fasicular reentry are usually associated with baseline conduction disease, including bundle branch block of either right or left and prolonged AV or PR interval, with the absence of such on a resting 12 lead ECG making them very unlikely to be the mechanism for the VT.

Scar Mediated Ventricular Tachycardia

Within westernized cultures the most common underlying cause of recurrent VT is remote coronary disease. Secondary to a focus on shorter door to balloon times for the acute myocardial infarction patient, more patients are surviving their myocardial infarctions only to eventually experience downstream congestive heart failure and ventricular tachycardia. The ischemic insult of a myocardial infarction results in the formation of myocardial scarring with variable transmural extent and resulting in altered electrical conduction within the infarcted myocardial region. Electrical conduction through scar is delayed and the resultant zone of slow conduction represents one of the critical elements of the reentrant circuit. This along with differential refractory periods in the surrounding tissue comprise the necessary substrate to sustain VT [5]. Ventricular ectopy is often the inciting event that initiates the ventricular tachyarrhythmia, either VT or VF. Premature ventricular contractions are sent through the slow conduction zone present within the ventricular scar with sufficient delay to result in their exit on the opposite side of the scarred region, finding the myocardium ready for depolarization. The electrical wave propagates around the more dense areas of scarring or anatomical barrier, such as heart valve annulus, and back into the entrance of the zone of slow conduction through the scar, creating a figure of eight pattern with the critical isthmus representing the central portion of the figure of eight (Fig. 7.4).

The typical ischemic ventricular tachycardia patient will present to medical care with either recurrent defibrillator therapies (shocks) or recurrent presyncope. Presyncope VT patients are often being treated with antitachycardia pacing and thus being prevented from progressing to either shocks or actual syncope. Of concern is the patient that presents with incessant VT or frequent - defined as >3 episodes of VT within 24 hours. This is termed VT storm and often requires multiple shocks and acute inpatient admission for management, accompanied by a significant rise in both inpatient and short term mortality [6]. The management of all of these patients is similar with a few exceptions made for the VT storm patient. In general, recurrent antitachycardia pacing or lone outpatient ICD shocks should result in the initiation or acceleration of antiarrhythmic drug therapy, starting with sotalol or amiodarone, followed by the addition of mexiletine if necessary. It is also important to make sure that these patients are adequately beta blocked since the majority of

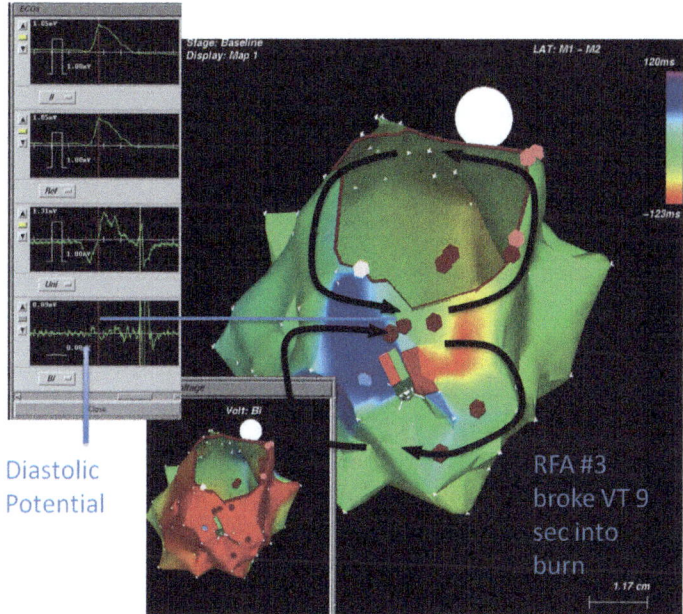

Diastolic
Potential

RFA #3
broke VT 9
sec into
burn

FIGURE 7.4 Figure of eight reentrant ventricular tachycardia circuit encircling around a dense inferoposterior left ventricular scar and the mitral valve annulus. The central portion of the figure of eight comprises the critical isthmus with a zone of slow conduction and the area where diastolic potentials may be recorded. This site, following confirmation with pacing maneuvers, often is the target of successful ablation

ischemic VT's are going to possess an adrenergic component and be beneficially treated with beta blockade. Once patients experience recurrent ICD therapies for VT while on an appropriate antiarrhythmic drug regimen, ventricular tachycardia ablation should be considered.

The management of VT storm patients is more difficult and varied than the ambulatory ischemic cardiomyopathy patient with recurrent ATP or lone ICD shocks for ventricular tachycardia. VT storm patients who present with recurrent ICD shocks often are accompanied by hemodynamic instability. The first step in their management is to establish control of their ventricular rhythm. Intravenous antiarrhythmic agents are utilized acutely to achieve this with both amiodarone and lidocaine used commonly. Although limited by toxicity, lidocaine can be a useful agent especially if there are concerns for ongoing ischemia. However, a combination of amiodarone (or sotalol) and lidocaine is often required to achieve control of the malignant ventricular arrhythmias in this situation. In addition to antiarrhythmic drug therapy and aggressive beta blockade, sedation and sometimes intubation are utilized to minimize adrenergic contribution to the VT. As an illustrative point to the contribution of sympathetic tone to the generation of recurrent VT in patients with an abnormal LVEF, bilateral sympathectomy has been recently shown to be effective for the suppression of acute ICD therapies for VT storm patients and has displayed durability over medium term follow up [7].

Following the initiation of intravenous antiarrhythmic drug therapy, ongoing myocardial ischemia should be considered and evaluated, likely with coronary angiography. If myocardial ischemia is present and is the main substrate of the VT, successful treatment with revascularization often subsides the VT. However, it is usually required to accelerate the patient's oral antiarrhythmic drug therapy prior to discharge and to establish short term follow up to make sure that the treated lesion was indeed the ischemic driver of the VT.

For VT storm patients or ambulatory patients with recurrent VT despite antiarrhythmic drug therapy, electrophysiologic testing and ablation of their VT should be considered. VT ablation has evolved since its inception to a well defined repeatable process designed to identify electrical scar, the culprit ventricular tachycardia and its dependent isthmus.

Electrophysiologic Evaluation of VT with Structural Heart Disease

For patients being evaluated for EP testing and ablation of a ventricular arrhythmia it is important to provide the appropriate setting. The use of general anesthesia for these procedures has become standard secondary to the length of the procedure and the risk for multiple defibrillations. Three dimensional mapping systems have also become standard and represent one of the most powerful tools to allow an in depth study of the ventricular chamber in question and increase the efficacy of VT ablation.

Prior to the procedure, the patient should be thoroughly assessed regarding the appropriate approach to the chamber in question. Generally the right ventricle does not pose much of a challenge outside of patients with complex congenital heart disease or tricuspid valve surgery. However, the left ventricle may prove inaccessible from a retroaortic or trans-septal approach due to the presence of mechanical aortic or mitral valves. The location of culprit scar is also an important consideration as posterior, inferior and lateral scars are more easily accessible from a transseptal approach while LVOT, and anterior and septal scars are via a retroaortic approach. Peripheral arterial disease can make a retro aortic approach difficult if not impossible, which should prompt the perfor-mance of a peripheral arterial exam (bruits and pulses) prior to procedure onset. In addition, the ability to access the epi-cardial space (the absence of a prior sternotomy) should also be considered at procedure onset to determine if it is an option if required.

During procedure onset and throughout the duration, con-trol of the patient's bradyarrhythmia should be available through the implanted device (in the likely event that it is present). It is best to leave patients that are not ventricular pacing dependent paced in the atrium only to allow intrinsic conduction for more accurate endocardial scar mapping. For ventricular pacing dependent patients it is often necessary to leave biventricular pacing in place to maintain appropriate hemodynamic status for the purpose of anesthesia. It may also be necessary to review the induced ventricular tachycar-dia on the far field electrogram through the device, which is only possible if the programmer is on and communicating with the device. The implanted device can also provide a means of intracardiac defibrillation if such a rescue is needed.

Once access to the LV endocardium or epicardium has been obtained, electrophysiologic study and ablation of ventricular tachycardia proceeds in five steps: (1) anatomic definition; (2) endocardial scar mapping; (3) induction and study of ventricular tachycardia, including entrainment mapping; (4) ablation of ventricular tachycardia, late potentials within scar; (5) attempt reinduction of ventricular tachycardia. With abolition of the clinical ventricular tachycardia and inability to induce anything other than ventricular fibrillation (rate >200 bpm) the study is complete.

To define the left ventricular anatomy a three dimensional map is generated with the aid of either fluoroscopy or ultrasound, and often both. Other than the geometry of the left ventricle itself, this often includes structures such as the mitral annulus, left ventricular outflow tract, left sided His bundle, Purkinje potentials and papillary muscles. It is important to make sure that the anatomy collected is complete. Correspondingly, the right ventricular structures including the AV node and the His conduction system, tricuspid valve, pulmonic valve, right ventricular outflow tract should be noted. Generally the risk of right ventricular perforation is higher and thus more care during mapping is needed. As the definition of endocardial scarring is dependent upon catheter contact with the wall, it is essential to know if contact is indeed present; otherwise areas will be labeled as scar inappropriately. This has been aided with real time two dimensional intracardiac echocardiography along with the evolution of contact force catheters, both of which can be used to provide definitive evidence of endocardial contact. Multi electrode mapping catheters are commonly utilized to collect a significantly larger amount of data in a shorter period of time both regarding anatomy and endocardial voltage.

Generally at the same time that anatomic information is collected, voltage is collected to provide visual information of the distribution of endocardial scarring relative to the anatomy collected. The definition of endocardial scar varies somewhat but is generally accepted to be any myocardial tissue with less than 0.5 mv. In similar fashion to the necessity of complete anatomic collection, it is just as important to

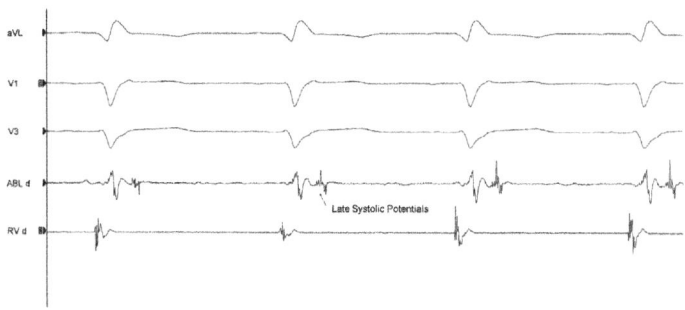

FIGURE 7.5 Late systolic potentials noted during substrate ventricular mapping recorded in sinus rhythm

generate a complete detailed voltage map. With identification of the scar, additional focus should be placed upon the scar itself for either fragmented potentials or late potentials most recently coined to be late areas of ventricular activation or LAVA. LAVA are characterized by high frequency or fragmented signals that can be either late relative to the QRS complex and local signal or buried completely within the local signal (Fig. 7.5).

In addition, areas that LV capture may be generated from within the endocardial scar are suspicious for possible VT isthmus and should be tagged for eventual ablation.

With a complete endocardial scar map, the next step within our lab is to induce ventricular tachycardia via programmed stimulation via a quadripolar pacing catheter in the RV. A predominantly substrate based approach does not involve induction of VT and ablation is carried out with the intention to abolish all LAVA within and around the endocardial scar. At this point it is crucial to reference the tachycardia 12-lead ECG for the rate and appearance of the VT, if available. Within the defibrillator population one may not ever have a surface electrocardiogram as the majority of their events are treated prior to presentation to medical care via their device. As a result only the cycle length and far field electrogram through the device are available to correlate the VT induced during the procedure with the clinical VT.

Once VT is induced matching the clinical VT the approach to study of the VT can vary from patient to patient. If the VT is hemodynamically tolerable (most often seen with slower VT's [<150 bpm] in patients with only moderate LV dysfunction) then activation and entrainment mapping may be pursued. If not hemodynamically tolerable, then the VT is pace terminated or terminated via defibrillation and pace mapping to define the VT isthmus based upon the VT morphology followed by a LAVA ablation strategy is appropriate. Both situations will be discussed in the following sections.

The Study of Hemodynamically Tolerable VT

Hemodynamically tolerable VT has become increasingly uncommon within the electrophysiology lab. Most of the VT's that are being mapped currently are fast VT's in patients with more advanced LV dysfunction. It may often be necessary to utilize vasopressors or in some cases device based hemodynamic support (Intra-aortic balloon pump, percutaneous left ventricular assist device such as Impella or ECMO) to provide adequate perfusion pressure in an effort to allow mapping. Goal blood pressures should be a mean arterial pressure above 50 mmHg.

When VT is tolerable it is beneficial to perform activation and entrainment mapping to confidently abolish the clinical VT. Points are taken and recorded via the mapping system to identify early and late EGM's with the area in the scar connecting early to late representing the slow component of the VT circuit and the critical isthmus. Within the early meets late area entrainment via the mapping catheter is performed by pacing 10–20 ms faster than the VT. Capture is maintained for sufficient time to overtake the VT circuit (5–10 beats) followed by cessation. If the morphology of the tachycardia changes during pacing, termed "manifest entrainment", and is associated with a post pacing interval (PPI) longer than the tachycardia cycle length then the pacing site is from an area outside of the tachycardia circuit. Ablation at these sites will not result in termination of VT. Suitable targets for successful

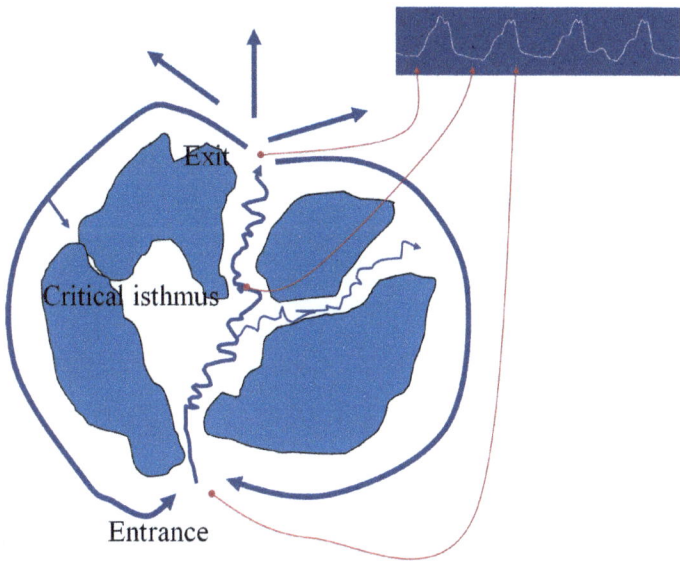

FIGURE 7.6 Diagram illustrating VT circuit with entrance, exit and critical isthmus sites denoted

ablation should results in "concealed entrainment". Pacing from these sites results in acceleration and exact morphology match as the tachycardia. Sites associated with the highest short and long term success in eliminating the VT circuit with ablation are in the critical isthmus. In addition to concealed entrainment, pacing from within the critical isthmus, the difference between the PPI and the tachycardia cycle length (TCL) will be small (likely less than 20 ms), and recording of presystolic potentials with an activation time to surface QRS similar to stimulus to surface QRS (also less than 20 ms) indicate that the mapping catheter is located within the VT critical isthmus (Fig. 7.6).

Ablation at this site typically at 30–45 W with an irrigated ablation catheter should result in the termination of VT promptly (Figs. 7.7, 7.8, and 7.9).

In some cases the isthmus is wide and some catheter manipulation is required to completely transect the isthmus.

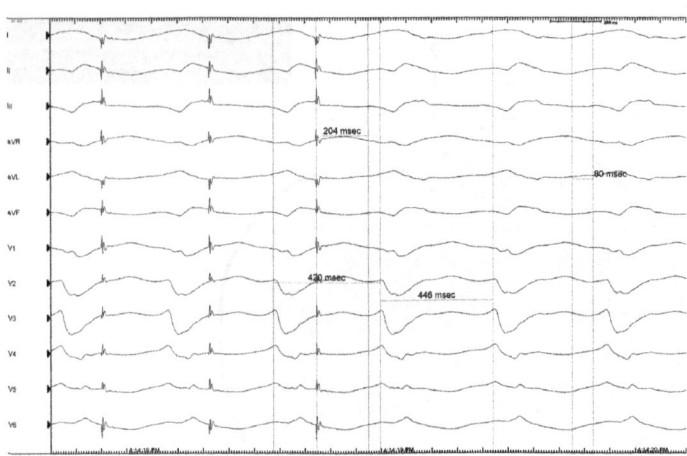

FIGURE 7.7 Pacing from the critical isthmus of the VT circuit resulting in "concealed entrainment" with 12 out of 12 lead surface ECG match in pacing morphology as compared with VT morphology

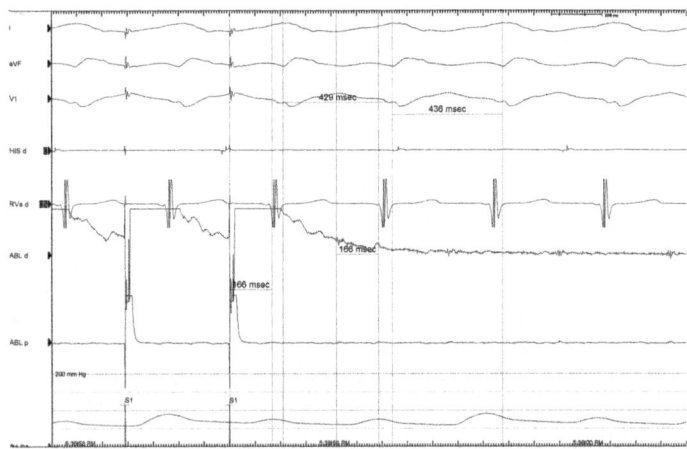

FIGURE 7.8 Other criteria for pacing within the critical isthmus of the VT circuit with pacing stimulus to QRS = EGM to QRS and post pacing interval (PPI) roughly equal to VT cycle length

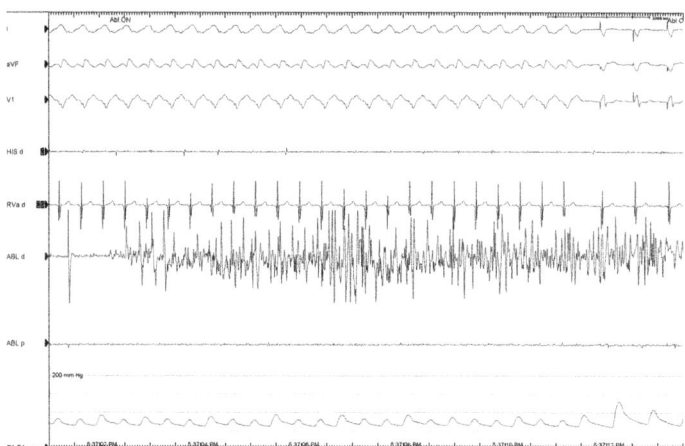

FIGURE 7.9 Ablation at the critical isthmus site results in termination of VT

Following thorough ablation of the isthmus (noncapture of the targeted region with high output pacing via the mapping catheter), the culprit VT should be rendered non-inducible. Once found to be non-inducible, scar modification via targeting of LAVA is usually undertaken to improve the long term success of the VT ablation and hopefully prevent subsequent VT's. This approach will be discussed in the third and final study/ablation approach.

The Study of Hemodynamically Unstable VT

Induction of hemodynamically unstable VT should be followed by termination of the VT either via pacing or defibrillation. The VT is then reviewed with the vector of the VT QRS utilized to identify the exit site from the identified endocardial scar. At this stage, pace mapping to the induced VT with a software based approach typically provided through the 3D mapping system is used to identify the exit (best match, generally >90 % in 12 leads, ideally >95 % match) and entrance (worst match) with the isthmus connecting the two. Entrance and exit are usually spatially related as the length of the typical VT isthmus is usually 20–30 mm and with detailed pace mapping can be readily identified. This isthmus is transsected with thorough ablation rendering the targeted area not able to be captured with pacing and the VT should be rendered noninducible. Following abolition of the clinical VT additional scar modification is generally performed similar to that following successful entrainment and activation guided VT ablation.

Scar Modification for VT

Scar modification or homogenization has been utilized as a primary approach for patients with unstable VT's or multiple VT's and is often performed after successful abolition of the culprit clinical VT. With detailed scar mapping, LAVA are targeted with the goal of elimination of the late potential. A more diffuse approach can also be taken where the entire scar is ablated, or linear transsecting lesions are placed through the scar, or the scar is circumscribed with contiguous ablation. Areas with the ability to capture the LV within the scar are also common targets for scar modification. The major downside of this as a primary approach is the uncertainty regarding successful treatment of the culprit clinical VT. Of the strategies available, LAVA, linear lesions, abolition of pacing capture or scar isolation, the selected strategy is often dependent upon the location and size of the scar accompanied by the comfort level of the performing physician. Recent data supports favorable results following LAVA guided scar homogenization; however, it is not always possible to completely eliminate every LAVA within the scar which may make the use of a more diffuse strategy an appropriate backup measure.

Epicardial Mapping

Often when one is unable to successfully eradicate the culprit VT via endocardial mapping and ablation, the consideration of epicardial mapping follows. It is important to consider this option when discussing the procedure with the patient to make sure that the risks of this approach are understood. Prior cardiac surgery makes this significantly more difficult and should serve as a relative contraindication to this approach.

Our approach is to obtain epicardial access via a dry pericardial tap; a subxyphoid approach is generally utilized with the area prepped and draped as per routine to start. A Tuohy needle is utilized and advanced slowly under the sternum staying as anterior as possible under fluoroscopy. The glide wire present within the needle can be advanced intermittently to see if the needle has found the pericardial space. Once the wire enters the pericardial space it should be advanced aggressively to wrap the entire outline of the pericardium in multiple loops. Once the wire is in place a short steerable epicardial sheath is advanced over the wire into the pericardial space. Following this, anatomic and voltage/scar mapping using a multi electrode or ablation catheter can proceed in the same fashion as endocardial mapping. Entrainment and pace mapping can be performed similar to the endocardium as well with the major limiting factor being the ability to capture the LV due to the presence of epicardial fat in areas. It is always important to define coronary anatomy via coronary angiography with the ablation catheter in the area of desired ablation prior to ablation in an effort to not directly ablate a major epicardial vessel. Once the scar has been mapped and the isthmus defined to be within a safe region, ablation is generally performed at 25–35 W via an irrigated ablation catheter.

With a complete ablation within the pericardium a pigtail drain is exchanged for the steerable sheath over wire with the drain left in place overnight. Prior to removal of the drain, our practice is to infuse corticosteroids (either Solumedrol or hydrocortisone) within the pericardial space to minimize the risk of subsequent pericarditis.

Electrophysiologic Evaluation of Idiopathic VT

There is a well-defined category of VT seen in patients who are typically younger without structural or ischemic cardio-vascular disease. Outflow tract VT's and high volume PVC's are the predominant arrhythmias encountered within this category. These normal heart VT's may originate from the outflow tract and some originate from the inferoposterior septal LV, termed as fascicular or "Belhassen" variant VT. It is important to have a clinical suspicion for these less common VT's as the procedural approach to their electrophysi-ologic study and treatment is quite different from VT with structural cardiovascular disease. VT's originating from the outflow tracts typically have an inferior axis with large R wave amplitudes in the inferior leads (Fig. 7.10).

The morphology of the idiopathic inferoposterior septal LV VT is consistent with typical right bundle branch block pattern with an LAFB axis (Fig. 7.11).

Outflow tract VT's, especially those originating from the right ventricular regions, are well understood to be due to triggered activity and are generally responsive to beta block-ade and calcium channel blockade medical therapy. On the other hand, fasicular or "Belhassen VT" has also been coined "Verapamil Sensitive VT" because its mechanism is thought be due to a small circuit reentry in the inferoposterior septum that is calcium dependent. Often invasive electrophysiologic study and ablation are reserved for medical treatment failures with these agents.

For patients with symptomatic idiopathic PVC's, the majority of the clinical decision making centers around the

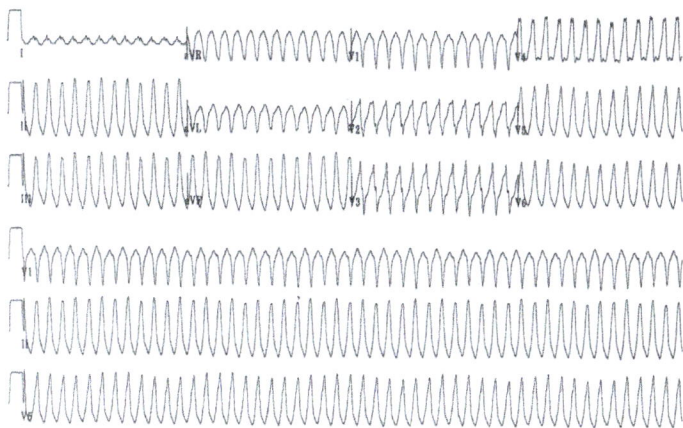

FIGURE 7.10 Twelve lead ECG of a patient with ventricular tachycardia originating from the right ventricular outflow tract. Note the typical left bundle branch block morphology with inferior QRS axis as well as the large R wave amplitudes in the inferior leads

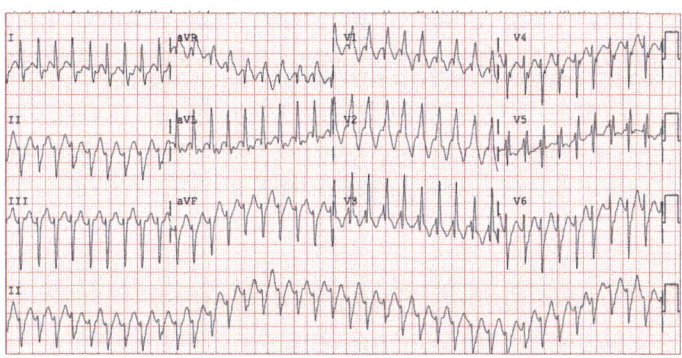

FIGURE 7.11 Twelve lead ECG of a patient with an idiopathic normal heart ventricular tachycardia originating from the left ventricular inferoposterior septum. Note the right bundle branch block morphology with superior QRS axis

burden of PVC's and their location. A PVC burden of at least 10 % or greater on ambulatory monitoring is considered high volume and at risk for developing subsequent PVC induced LV dysfunction. PVC origins within the RVOT are lowest risk for PVC cardiomyopathy with any LV location being higher risk for downstream LV functional decline. In addition, PVC's with a QRS duration of greater than 150 ms are also high risk for LV dyssynchrony and if frequent enough volume can cause LV dysfunction.

Medical therapy via beta blockade alone often may result in some reduction in the PVC burden, but some patients may still be left with high volume PVC's and at risk for car-diomyopathy even on medical therapy. Antiarrhythmic drug therapy via Class 1 (flecainide, propafenone, mexiletine) or Class III (sotalol, amiodarone) may result in a further reduction in PVC burden which may be utilized as adjunc-tive therapy for patients with high volume PVC's. Once on medical therapy, PVC burden should be reassessed with repeat ambulatory monitoring to make sure that the PVC burden on therapy is low enough to preclude the develop-ment of PVC induced cardiomyopathy. Persistence of high volume PVC's or symptoms despite antiarrhythmic drug therapy should prompt consideration for electrophysiologic study and ablation of the PVC focus. The presence of multi-form PVC's or non-outflow tract locations are risk factors for requiring multiple procedures to effectively reduce the PVC burden and should be discussed with the patient prior to proceeding.

Electrophysiologic Testing and Ablation of Idiopathic PVC's and Outflow Tract VT's

After medical treatment failure or in patients unwilling to attempt medical therapy, electrophysiologic testing with an eye to ablation therapy for those with documented outflow tract VT or high volume idiopathic PVC's is appropriate. Of note, these procedures generally do not require general anesthesia and are best approached with as little sedation as possible secondary to a reduction in PVC burden associated with aggressive sedation. Without spontaneous PVC's it is difficult to confidently map and eliminate the PVC. Isuprel, atropine, aminophylline and programmed stimulation from either the RV apex or outflow tract are often utilized. Generally outflow tract patients have single outflow tract PVC's that represent the source of their more sustained episodes of VT. Mapping and ablation of these PVC's usually treats their sustained VT. For PVC patients it is important to determine their triggers. If their PVC's come out when they are resting, sedation may be appropriate; in contrast, if they are associated with caffeine, aminophylline may be appropriate, etc.

The PVC morphology is captured once the patient is on the table and logged within the 3D mapping system for comparison should pace mapping be utilized. Usually QRS morphology can be used to identify location of the PVC (LVOT or RVOT) with the precordial transition being the most useful but imperfect tool. R/S transition prior to V3 can confidently be labeled as LVOT with a transition after V3 labeled as RVOT. The use of multielectrode mapping catheters for anatomic, pacing and activation mapping can make identification of the PVC focus easier. Once in the appropriate location anatomy is collected, first with particular attention to details such as the His bundle on the RV side and the aortic cusp/coronary anatomy on the LV side. Ultrasound can be of great use for aortic and LVOT PVC's/VT to minimize the risk of damage to sensitive structures such as the ostium of the left or right coronary arteries.

With anatomy collected, the preferential modality is activation mapping of spontaneous PVC's focusing on only including PVC's that are completely consistent with the clinical PVC and not catheter induced. Once the area of activation is narrowed down sufficiently the exact area should be able to be identified usually with a small pre potential prior to the larger local EGM on the mapping or ablation catheter. Favorable ablation sites usually have a pre potential or EGM onset of 35 ms or greater ahead of the surface QRS complex. When mapping in the RVOT provides no significantly early sites of activation, consideration of LV mapping should be undertaken prior to ablating. Pace mapping with software guided matching can be used to successfully locate infrequent PVC's within the EP lab (albeit with a somewhat lower success rate) and/or confirm the best site identified via activation mapping.

Electrophysiologic Study and Ablation of Idiopathic LVVT's

Idiopathic reentrant LVVT's make up less than 5 % of the LVVT's encountered in general electrophysiologic practice (with the majority being ischemic, outflow tract or high volume PVC's). However, their behavior and treatment differs such that they are deserving of special interest. With the electrocardiographic characteristics discussed previously, it is important to have a high index of suspicion dependent upon the resting and tachycardia ECG going into the invasive electrophysiologic study. During EP study it is important to induce the VT with a morphology that is consistent with the clinical VT. Entrainment from the inferoposterior septum of the left ventricle generally provides a favorable PPI-TCL, with entrainment from the atrium remaining possible but usually showing a less favorable PPI-TCL.

Ablation of this rhythm is usually accomplished through targeting of Purkinjie potentials along the distal LV apex via a retroaortic (or transseptal) approach. Purkinjie potentials are sharp high voltage fragmented signals distal to the LBBB. Radiofrequency energy applied at this point with an ablation catheter often would terminate the tachycardia and render the VT non-inducible. With a loss of tachycardia inducibility the procedure is terminated and deemed successful.

VT of Special Consideration, Bundle Branch Reentry

Bundle branch reentry VT is a rare but important subtype of VT. These are mostly observed in patients with dilated cardiomyopathy with underlying conduction disease. When suspicious of BBRVT, it is important to remember that BBRVT typically uses the diseased bundle branch (present on the resting 12 lead ECG and typically the left bundle branch) as the antegrade conducting limb of the circuit with the healthy limb as the retrograde limb. An important clue to bundle branch reentry VT is presentation of tachycardia that displays the same QRS morphology at baseline but with findings of atrio-ventricular dissociation (Figs. 7.12 and 7.13).

Entrainment from the right ventricular apex usually results in a favorable PPI when compared to the tachycardia cycle length. It is usually possible to entrain the arrhythmia from the atrium given the necessary participation of the His-Purkinjie system in the tachycardia, but with a long PPI relative to the tachycardia cycle length. As atrial activation is usually retrograde and thus dependent upon the reentrant circuit distal to the His bundle, changes in atrial cycle length are preceded by changes in the ventricular tachycardia cycle length. BBRVT typically has a morphology consistent with a full bundle branch block either left or more commonly right bundle branch block.

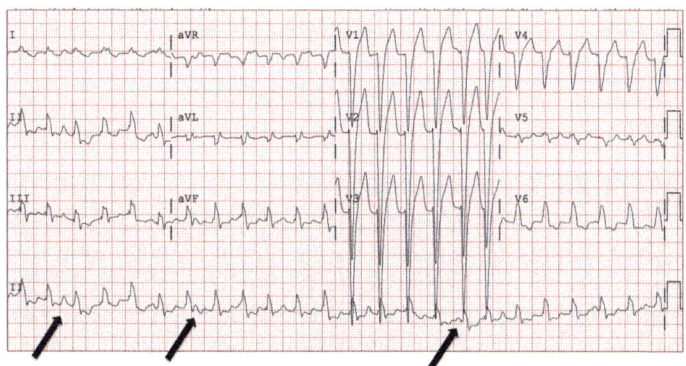

FIGURE 7.12 Twelve lead ECG of a patient with Bundle Branch Reentry VT. The *arrows* denote p waves with dissociation of atrial (p waves) and ventricular (QRS signals) signals

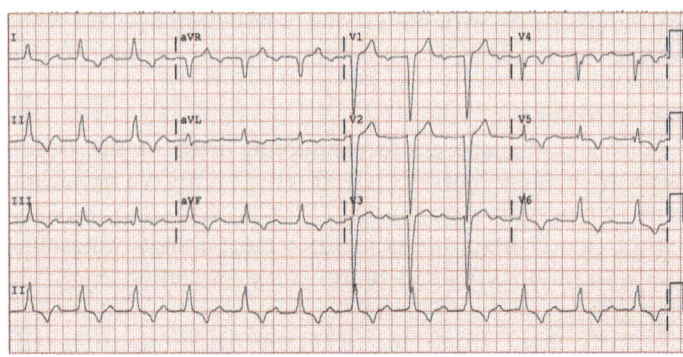

FIGURE 7.13 Baseline 12 lead ECG of the same patient with bundle branch reentry VT during sinus rhythm. Note with exact same QRS morphology in sinus rhythm as during VT

The ablation of this arrhythmia generally surrounds targeting the involved bundle branch with an ablation catheter, often during the induced ventricular tachycardia. Termination of the VT to sinus rhythm and loss of inducibility are appropriate endpoints for deeming the procedure successful and result in its termination. The right bundle potential is usually found apically to the His bundle on the septum. If the ablation catheter is positioned appropriately the right bundle potential can be separated from the His signal with a slight additional apical extension required to safely ablate the bundle branch and avoid the His bundle.

Mapping Considerations

When mapping idiopathic VT in 3D, most commonly the window of interest will be set to capture the PVCs that spontaneously occur throughout the procedure. In some rare instances in which the patient can hemodynamically tolerate the VT, a faster map can be acquired. Most of the time, however, a map will be constructed that acquires electroanatomic (EA) data only on the spontaneous PVC locations.

Anatomy is always a concern when mapping PVCs, especially in the outflow tracts, due to the way the ventricle contracts on a PVC. Continuous acquisition of anatomy during RS can confuse the picture while mapping. While it is a slower process, it may be better to take a traditional "point by point" map on the 3D mapping system (Biosene Webster's Carto system can take point by point, rather than continuous, anatomy). This way, the entire map is built as a PVC map, rather than as a mix of NSR and PVCs. Another way to acquire a consistent anatomy is to use the CartoSound mapping technology. Each ultrasound contour can be taken only on PVCs, so that a quick PVC-only anatomy can be built; EA data can then be plotted on the CartoSound map.

The key to setting a window of interest and mapping is to make sure only ventricular activation is being annotated. Points acquired by the tricuspid or mitral valve will have both atrial and ventricular signals. It is also important to be certain the points acquired are all in the intrinsic PVC, and not on a catheter-induced or clinically irrelevant PVC. This can become complicated when a patient presents with multiple morphologies of their PVC. It is usually best to try to map one PVC at a time, rather than constantly toggling between maps and risking missing beats.

Another difficulty with mapping and treating PVCs is frequency on the day of procedure. A wide variety of factors, including strength of sedation, can play a role in how many PVCs a patient has during a procedure. Electrophysiologists are often frustrated to see a large PVC burden on a holter monitor, only to have the PVCs go silent or occur only rarely during a procedure. In these instances, pace-mapping is often performed, with varying results. Traditionally this has been difficult to map and very time-consuming. Because the matching of a paced morphology to the intrinsic PVC is subjective, the best the operator and EA mapper can usually do is determine the best matches (usually placed on a scale with the 12 leads, e.g., "This is an 11/12 match") and mark these spots anatomically on the 3D map.

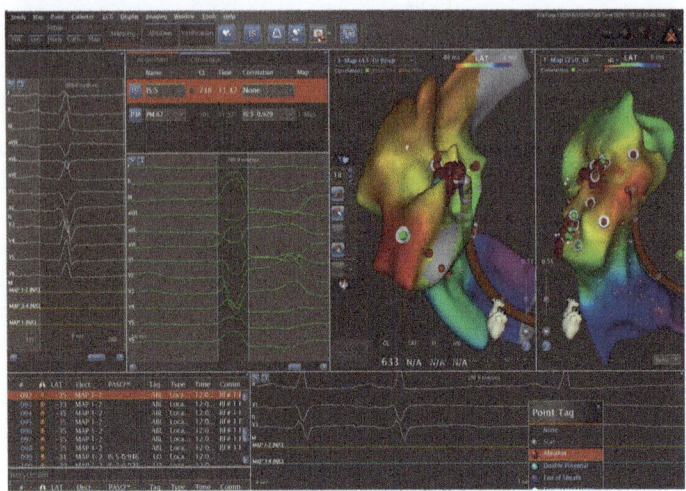

FIGURE 7.14 Paso Technology (Biosense Webster, Diamond Bar, CA). Pacemap points are tagged as *green* or *red* and given a percentage match to intrinsic PVC. Ablation strategy is targeted toward highest percentage pace map matches when intrinsic PVCs occur rarely

More recently, however, 3D mapping technology has advanced to make this process faster and more accurate. PASO software from Biosense Webster now allows the user to store the intrinsic PVC, or store multiple intrinsic PVCs, and then automatically tags and colors the map based on a percentage match to the various intrinsic PVCs (e.g., This is a 97 % match to the intrinsic PVC). This allows the electrophysiologist to pace-map multiple morphologies at a time (Fig. 7.14).

Mapping ischemic VT has its own unique challenges. Like with idiopathic VT, it is rare to map activation during VT, due to hemodynamic instability. Because VT that comes from ischemia is usually reentrant, in the rare case that activation mapping is performed, the window of interest should be set at 90 % of the cycle length, with a distinct, sharp peak of a body surface ECG lead as the "time zero" reference point.

Usually, however, substrate mapping will be performed. Setting the window of interest for mapping ischemic substrate is not complicated, but it is critical to get it right. Rather than collecting timing, the map will collect and represent bipolar voltage. Usually a scale of 0.5–1.5 mv is set – this makes everything below 0.5 mv to be considered dense scar, and everything above 1.5 mv to be considered healthy tissue. Everything between 0.5 and 1.5 mv is then displayed on a color scale representing various levels of tissue health. This color scale between 0.5 and 1.5 mv will usually show up on the "border zone" of dense scar. With a high density map, electrophysiologists will also be able to find channels of viable tissue through the dense scar, which helps locate the zones of slow conduction through the scar responsible for the reentrant tachycardias. Close attention should be paid to fragmented electrograms and late potentials, as these also represent zones of slow conduction through scar areas. Pace-map matching software can also be used to identify the critical isthmus for ischemic VT. If the VT is induced or observed during the procedure, the morphology can be saved in Paso, and pacing can be performed through scar areas to identify VT match (Figs. 7.15 and 7.16).

Substrate mapping can be problematic when careful attention is not applied to the acquired points. The points should be consistent. Mapping in SR is preferable, but not always possible. When mapping in SR, the 3D mapper must be careful only to take sinus points; paced beats or catheter-induced PVCs should be discarded. When mapping a paced ventricle, the window of interest must be set to exclude the pacing spike which will be present on the mapping catheter. If the window does not exclude this pacing spike, the map will confuse it with an actual electrogram. The most important, basic rule while mapping a substrate: anything inside the window is "seen" and measured as voltage by the mapping system! Be sure to exclude anything that is not intrinsic EGM.

A final difficulty to overcome when substrate mapping is the anatomical challenge of the left ventricle. Large papillary muscles, chordae tendonae, and trabeculation are all

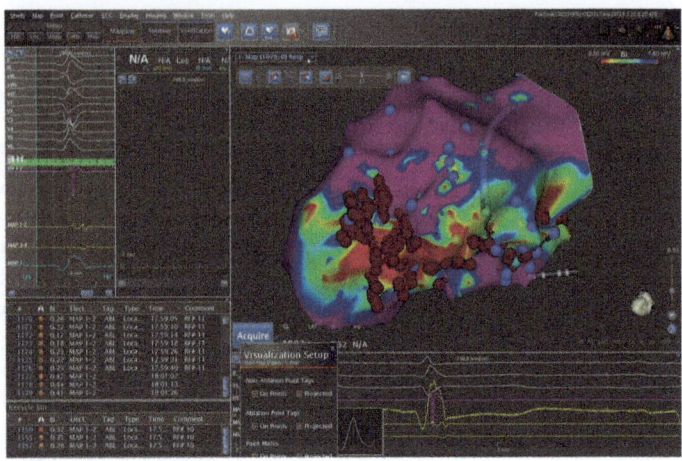

FIGURE 7.15 3D substrate map of ischemic VT. *Red areas* are dense scar (<0.5 mv). *Purple areas* are healthy tissue (>0.5 mv). *Yellow, green* and *blue* represent damaged "border zone" tissue. Ablation strategy here targeted a critical isthmus through the middle of the scar

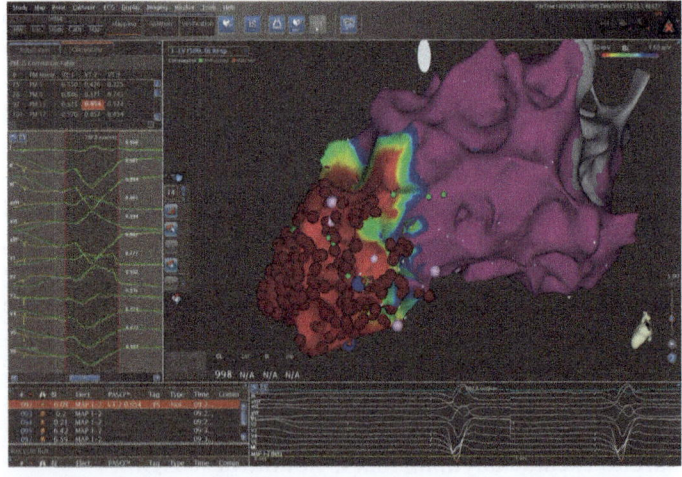

FIGURE 7.16 Paso technology in ischemic VT. Apical scar was targeted for extensive ablation. Paso revealed two channels (*small red dots* inside of dark blue tags), representing 95 % matches to two different VT morphologies. These VTs were non-inducible post-ablation

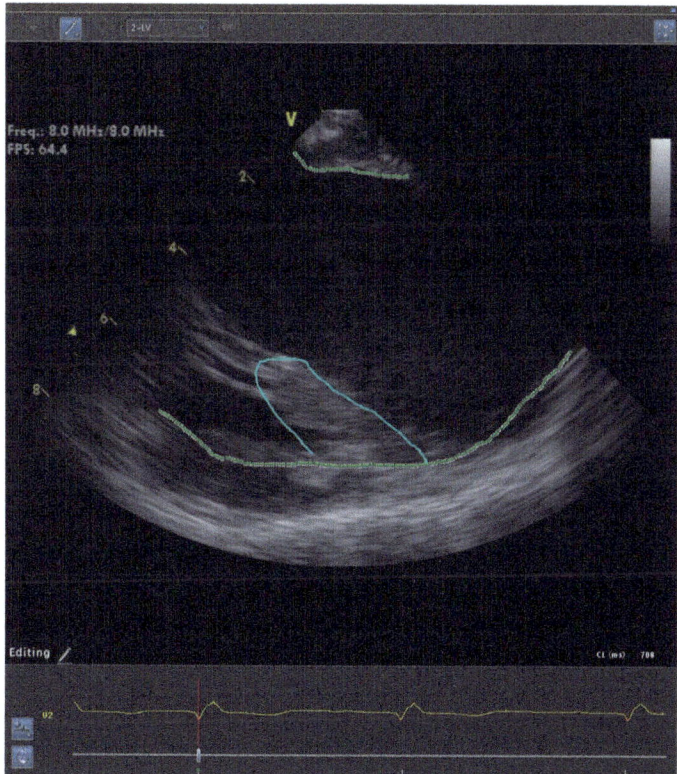

FIGURE 7.17 Papillary muscle drawn on the CartoSound technology. Papillary muscles are then represented in 3D on the map, so the catheter navigation and contact assessment can take these into account

anatomical challenges that make catheter maneuvering and mapping difficult. For this reason, phased array ICE is often used. When paired with CartoSound technology, the 3D map can actually display internal structures like papillary muscles, giving important knowledge for how to navigate and where to map (Fig. 7.17).

Additionally, with these internal structures, it can be hard to know whether or not the catheter is in good contact with the tissue. If the catheter does not have good contact, and a point is acquired, the map will read the lack of electrogram as dense scar. This can be misleading, plotting scar on the 3D map while the catheter is actually floating off the tissue. Contact force sensing technology can solve this problem. By measuring the actual contact and force of contact against the tissue, operators can know whether they are in contact with the tissue and apply consistent force of contact throughout the map. The confusion surrounding "internal" versus "real" points on a map is virtually eliminated with a contact force sensing catheter.

Summary

Ventricular tachyarrhythmias are an increasingly common occurrence with the growing ICD population. Knowledge of the electrophysiologic characteristics and treatment of these arrhythmias continues to grow. For the majority of these patients recurrences downstream are a constant risk and may require ongoing antiarrhythmic drug therapy for complete suppression. In experienced hands it is possible to study and treat these arrhythmias successfully in a safe fashion. However, as our knowledge of the benefit of VT ablation grows it is becoming increasingly clear that this procedure, when performed properly, can further reduce the risk of subsequent ICD shocks and mortality [8, 9].

References

1. Farzaneh-Far A, Lerman BB. Idiopathic ventricular outflow tract tachycardia. Heart. 2005;91(2):136–8.
2. Brugada P, Brugada J, Mont L, et al. A new approach to the differential diagnosis of a regular tachycardia with a wide QRS complex. Circulation. 1991;83:1649–59.
3. Vereckei A, Duray G, Szenasi G, et al. New algorithm using only lead aVR for differential diagnosis of wide QRS complex tachycardia. Heart Rhythm. 2008;5:89–98.

4. Pava LR, Perfan P, Badiel M, et al. R-wave peak time at DII: a new criterion for differentiating between wide complex QRS tachycardias. Heart Rhythm. 2010;7:922.
5. Stevenson WG, Friedman PL, Sager PT, et al. Exploring postinfarction reentrant ventricular tachycardia with entrainment mapping. J Am Coll Cardiol. 1997;29(6):1180–9.
6. Sesselberg HW, et al. Ventricular arrhythmia storms in postinfarction patients with implantable defibrillators for primary prevention indications: a MADIT-II substudy. Heart Rhythm. 2007;4(11):1395–402.
7. Vaseghi M, Gima J, Kanaan C, Ajijola OA, Marmureanu A, Mahajan A, Shivkumar K. Cardiac sympathetic denervation in patients with refractory ventricular arrhythmias or electrical-storm: intermediate and long-term follow-up. Heart Rhythm. 2014;11(3):360–6.
8. Reddy VY, et al. Prophylactic catheter ablation for the prevention of defibrillator therapy. N Engl J Med. 2007;357(26):2657–65.
9. Kuck KH, Schaumann A, Eckardt L, et al. Catheter ablation of stable ventricular tachycardia before defibrillator implantation in patients with coronary heart disease (VTACH): a multicentre randomised controlled trial. Lancet. 2010;375(9708):31–40.

Chapter 8
Hereditary Arrhythmias

Alon Barsheshet and Ilan Goldenberg

Ventricular tachyarrhythmias (ventricular tachycardia [VT] or ventricular fibrillation [VF]) are associated with syncope, aborted cardiac arrest (ACA) or sudden cardiac death (SCD). Patients will experience syncope, ACA, or SCD depending on the duration of the VT and whether VT deteriorates into VF.

The etiology of these life-threatening hereditary arrhythmias can be classified according to whether structural heart disease is present or not. Structural causes of hereditary arrhythmias include dilated cardiomyopathy, hypertrophic cardiomyopathy, and arrhythmogenic right ventricular

A. Barsheshet, MD (✉)
Cardiology Department, Rabin Medical Center,
Petah Tikva, Israel

Sackler Faculty of Medicine, Tel-Aviv University, Tel-Aviv, Israel

Cardiology Division, University of Rochester Medical Center,
Rochester, New York
e-mail: Barshesheta@gmail.com

I. Goldenberg, MD
Cardiology Department, The Leviev Heart Center,
Sheba Medical Center, Tel Hashomer, Israel

Sackler Faculty of Medicine, Tel-Aviv University, Tel-Aviv, Israel

Cardiology Division, University of Rochester Medical Center,
Rochester, New York

D.T. Huang, T. Prinzi (eds.), *Clinical Cardiac Electrophysiology in Clinical Practice*, In Clinical Practice,
DOI 10.1007/978-1-4471-5433-4_8,
© Springer-Verlag London 2015

cardiomyopathy/dysplasia (ARVC/D). Most of the nonstructural causes of hereditary arrhythmias are cardiac channelopathies (disorders involving mutations in genes encoding cardiac ion channels) that include the congenital long QT syndromes (LQTS), Brugada syndrome, catecholaminergic polymorphic ventricular tachycardia (CPVT), and short QT syndrome.

This chapter will focus on the clinical and genetic aspects of the LQTS, Brugada syndrome, and ARVC/D. It should be noted that these genetic syndromes exhibit incomplete penetrance (i.e., the likelihood that a disease-causing mutation will have a phenotypic expression in a mutation-positive subject) and variable expressivity (i.e., different level of phenotypic expression), implicating environmental factors and possibly other genetic modifiers in the etiology of these diseases.

Long QT Syndrome

Incidence and Etiology

The long QT syndrome (LQTS) is a hereditary arrhythmia syndrome characterized by structurally normal heart and delayed ventricular repolarization as manifest on the ECG as abnormal QT interval prolongation.

Patients with LQTS are at an increased risk for sudden death resulting from episodes of VT, particularly torsades de point (polymorphic VT with a preceding long QT).

The estimated prevalence of LQTS is 1:2,000 of apparently healthy live-births [1]. About 85 % of the reported cases are inherited from one of the parents, with the remaining 15 % of affected patients having de novo mutations.

Two patterns of familial inheritance are predominant: autosomal dominant and autosomal recessive. The most common form is the autosomal dominant form, also called Romano-Ward syndrome.

The autosomal recessive form, also called Jervell-Lange-Nielsen syndrome, is a severe form of LQTS associated with congenital deafness.

To date, over 600 mutations have been recognized in 16 LQTS genes. LQT1, LQT2 and LQT3 account for 95 % of genotype-positive LQTS patients and about 75 % of all patients with LQTS [2].

Diagnosis and Classification

The diagnosis of LQTS is based on measurement of the corrected QT (QTc) on the ECG, clinical history, and/or genetic testing. A recent expert consensus statement [3] suggested that a diagnosis of LQTS can be made if one or more of the following criteria are fulfilled: (1) In the presence of a very prolonged QTc ($\geq$500 ms) in repeated 12-lead ECG and in the absence of a secondary cause for QT prolongation; (2) If a prolonged QTc is identified after a syncopal event in the absence of acquired causes of QT prolongation; (3) In the presence of an LQTS risk score (the Schwartz-Moss risk score based on personal and family history, symptomatology, and ECG) [4] $\geq$3.5; (4) In the presence of a pathogenic mutation in one of the LQTS genes.

It should be noted that about 25 % of patients with genetically confirmed LQTS exhibit QTc within normal range [5]. Four major provocative tests have been proposed to unmask LQTS patients with normal range QT at rest: (1) change from a supine to standing position [6], (2) during the recovery phase of exercise testing [7], (3) infusion of epinephrine [8], or (4) Adenosine-induced, sudden bradycardia and subsequent tachycardia [9].

LQTS is classified into 16 types according to the identified 16 LQTS associated genes with LQTS types 1–3 being the most common types of LQTS. LQTS type 1 accounts for 30–35 % of cases of LQTS and involves a loss of function mutation in the alpha subunit of the slow delayed rectifier potassium channel KCNQ1; the current through this channel is known as I_{Ks}.

LQTS type 2 accounts for 25–30 % of cases of LQTS and involves loss of function mutations in the alpha subunit of the rapid delayed rectifier potassium channel KCNH2 (or hERG); the current through this channel is known as I_{Kr}.

LQTS type 3 accounts for 5–10 % of cases of LQTS and involves a gain of function mutation in the alpha subunit of the sodium channel SCN5A, the current through this channel is known as I_{Na}.

LQTS types 4 through 14 are rare, each type accounts for less than 1 % of cases of LQTS. LQT5 involves a mutation in the beta subunit KCNE1 (or MinK) which co-assembles with KCNQ1. LQT6 involves a mutation in the beta subunit KCNE2 (or MiRP1) which co-assembles with KCNH2. LQT7 involves a mutation in the potassium channel gene KCNJ2; the current through this channel is called I_{K1}. It leads to Andersen-Tawil syndrome, which is associated with periodic paralysis and physical abnormalities including short stature, micrognathia, dental abnormalities, low-set ears, widely spaced eyes, and unusual curving of the fingers or toes (clinodactyly). LQT8 involves a mutation in the L type calcium channel encoded by the gene CACNA1c. It leads to Timothy's syndrome, which is associated with a very poor prognosis and also fusion of the fingers or toes (syndactily), flattened nose, small teeth, autism, and possible cardiac structural anomalies.

Genetic testing may have an important role in the diagnosis, risk stratification, and management of carriers of LQTS mutations. Currently, genetic testing is usually performed when there is a clinical suspicion of LQTS and for confirmatory testing among family members of identified probands.

Genotype-Phenotype Correlations and Risk Stratification

Genotype-phenotype correlation in the LQTS has been the most active line of research among the structurally normal heart diseases. It has been recognized that there is an association between the genetic background and clinical characteristics of the LQTS including electrocardiographic features, triggers for cardiac events, risk stratification and prognosis.

Moss et al. [10] have demonstrated that the ST-T wave repolarization pattern on the ECG differs among the 3 common LQTS genotypes. Patients with LQT1 typically have a broad-based T-wave pattern; patients with LQT2 exhibit a low amplitude bifid T-wave, whereas in LQT3, T-wave is usually peaked and late onset.

Importantly, cardiac events in LQTS were shown to be associated with gene-specific triggers. Patients with the LQT1

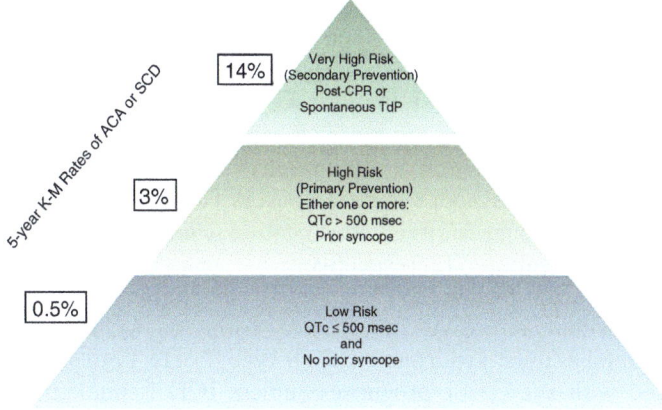

FIGURE 8.1 Suggested risk stratification for life threatening cardiac events in non- genotyped patients with the long QT syndrome. *ACA* aborted cardiac arrest, *KM* Kaplan Meier, *SCD* sudden cardiac death. The figure is taken with permission from reference[2]

genotype are at a higher risk for arrhythmic events triggered by sympathetic activation induced by exercise. Among the different types of exercise, swimming was shown to be a specific trigger for LQT1 patients [11, 12]. Patients with the LQT2 genotype are at a higher risk for arrhythmic events triggered by emotional stress, including anger, fear, startle, or sudden noise during sleep. Patients with the LQT3 genotype experience arrhythmic events mostly during sleep or at rest without emotional arousal.

Risk stratification among non-genotyped LQTS patients relies on a combined assessment of clinical and ECG factors. Figure 8.1 shows a suggested risk stratification scheme for non-genotyped patients with LQTS. Patients may be classified into three main risk categories: (1) The very high-risk group includes patients with a history of ACA and/or spontaneous torsades de pointes; these patients require an implantable cardioverter defibrillator (ICD) implantation for secondary prevention of SCD; (2) The high-risk group includes subjects with history of prior syncope or QTc > 500 ms, and (3) the low risk group includes those with QTc duration of ≤500 ms without prior syncope event [2].

Risk stratification among genotyped LQTS patients can be based on genotype-specific factors found to affect the phenotypic expression in patients with LQTS; those risk factors include age, gender, the post partum time period, menopause, prior syncope, mutation location, type of mutation (missense/non-missense), the biophysical function of the mutation and response to betablockers [13, 14]. Figures 8.2 and 8.3 show suggested risk stratification schemes for patients with LQT1 and LQT2, respectively.

The rare forms of LQTS Jervell-Lange-Nielsen syndrome (autosomal recessive inheritance form of LQTS) and Andersen-Tawil syndrome (LQTS type 7) are both associated with very poor prognoses (unless ICD is implanted); Patients with these syndromes experience life threatening arrhythmic events at an early age. Similarly, patients with multiple LQTS-associated mutations, particularly double mutations affecting the same gene, have been associated with a greater risk for life threatening arrhythmic events than patients who harbor a single mutation [15].

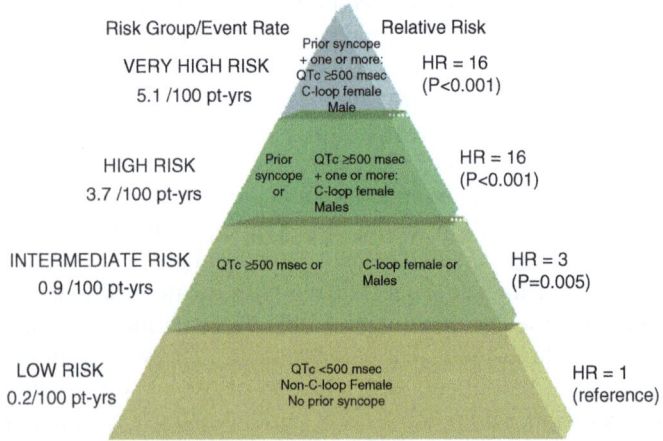

FIGURE 8.2 Proposed risk stratification for aborted cardiac arrest or sudden cardiac death in LQT1. *C-loop* mutations in cytoplasmic loops of the KCNQ1 channel, *Pt-yrs* patient years, *HR* hazard ratio. The figure is taken with permission from reference[47]

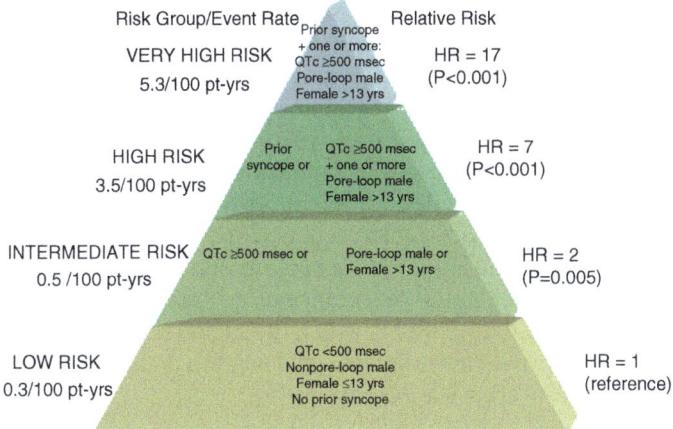

Risk Group/Event Rate		Relative Risk
VERY HIGH RISK 5.3/100 pt-yrs	Prior syncope + one or more: QTc ≥500 msec Pore-loop male Female >13 yrs	HR = 17 (P<0.001)
HIGH RISK 3.5/100 pt-yrs	Prior syncope or	QTc ≥500 msec + one or more Pore-loop male Female >13 yrs	HR = 7 (P<0.001)
INTERMEDIATE RISK 0.5 /100 pt-yrs	QTc ≥500 msec or	Pore-loop male or Female >13 yrs	HR = 2 (P=0.005)
LOW RISK 0.3/100 pt-yrs	QTc <500 msec Nonpore-loop male Female ≤13 yrs No prior syncope	HR = 1 (reference)

FIGURE 8.3 Proposed risk stratification scheme for aborted cardiac arrest or sudden cardiac death in LQT2 patients. *Pore-loop* muations in the pore-loop segments of the KCNH2 (hERG) channel, *Pt-yrs* patient years, *HR* hazard ratio. The figure is taken with permission from reference[14]

Management

In general, the treatment of LQTS consists of lifestyle modifications, medical therapy with beta-blockers, ICD and/or surgical therapy. The ACC/AHA/ESC guidelines [16] and a recently published expert consensus statement [3] recommend lifestyle modifications for all patients with a diagnosis of LQTS. Beta-blockers are recommended as a Class I indication for all patients with a clinical diagnosis of LQTS and as a Class IIa indication for patients with a genetic diagnosis of LQTS who have a normal QTc duration. Although there are limited data on the most effective dosage of beta-blockers, full dosing adjusted for age and weight is recommended. Abrupt discontinuation of beta-blockers should be avoided as this may cause exacerbation [3]. Implantation of an ICD is recommended for LQTS patients who experience an aborted cardiac arrest (class I indication) or for patients who had syncope and/or VT despite beta-blockers therapy (class IIa indication). The recently published expert consensus statement [3] recommends performing left cardiac sympathetic denervation (LCSD) in high-risk patients with a diagnosis of LQTS in whom ICD therapy is contraindicated or refused and/or beta-blockers are either not effective in preventing syncope/arrhythmias, not tolerated, or contraindicated (class I indication). In addition, the consensus statement has added that sodium channel blockers can be useful, as add-on therapy, for LQT3 patients with a QTc >500 ms who shorten their QTc by >40 ms following an acute oral sodium channel blocker test (class IIa indication) [3].

Lifestyle Modifications

The fact that patients with certain genotypes are more likely to experience their events under well-defined circumstances may provide insights into preventive measures. Patients with LQT1 have most of their events during exercise. Therefore, they should avoid strenuous exercise activity (particularly swimming) without supervision, and those at intermediate or high risk should not engage into competitive sports [3, 16]. Patients with LQT2 should be advised to avoid unexpected auditory stimuli as their cardiac events are predominantly associated with sudden arousal [17, 18]. Removal of loud noise stimuli at home and work such as elimination of alarm clocks, door bells and telephone ringing is usually recommended. LQT3 patients mainly experience events during sleep and at rest, and should be considered for a special intercom system in the bedroom. All patients with LQTS should avoid drugs known to prolong QT interval, or affect potassium and magnesium level. It is important to identify and correct electrolyte abnormalities that may occur during diarrhea, vomiting, metabolic conditions, or imbalanced diets for weight loss [3].

Beta-Blockers

Beta-blocker therapy is the mainstay treatment of patients with LQTS. The efficacy of this therapy in LQTS has been demonstrated in multiple studies. Moss et al. [19] have reported the efficacy of beta-blockers in 869 LQTS patients. Beta-blocker therapy was associated with a significant reduction in the rate of cardiac events in probands (0.97 ± 1.42 to 0.31 ± 0.86 events per year, $p < 0.001$) and in affected family members (0.26 ± 0.84 to 0.15 ± 0.69 events per year, $p < 0.001$). In another study among 549 LQT1 and 422 LQT2 patients from the International LQTS Registry, we have found that Beta-blocker therapy was associated with a prominent risk-reduction in high-risk patients, including a 67 % reduction ($P = 0.02$) in LQT1 males and a 71 % reduction ($P < 0.001$) in LQT2 females [20].

The protective effects of beta-blockers among LQTS patients may also depend on mutation location. We have shown among 860 patients with genetically confirmed LQT1 that beta-blocker therapy was associated with a significant 88 % reduction in the risk of life-threatening cardiac events among LQT1 carriers of the cytoplasmic loops (C-loop) missense mutations ($p = 0.02$), whereas among LQT1 carriers of non-C-loop missense mutations there was no significant reduction in the risk for life threatening cardiac events (HR 0.82, $p = 0.68$) [21]. It is known that the C-loops play an important role in the sympathetic regulation of the KCNQ1 channel [22]. Cellular expression studies have suggested that there is a combination of decrease in basal function and altered adrenergic regulation of the I_{Ks} channel in patients with C-loops missense mutations that may provide a potential explanation why beta-blockers are particularly effective in patients with this type of mutation [21].

The benefit associated with the various beta-blocker subtypes in the management of LQTS may not be equal. Two studies [20, 23] may suggest that metoprolol is less effective than Atenolol, Nadolol or Propranolol among LQT1 and LQT2 patients.

Potassium Supplementation

Potassium supplementation and spironolactone were proposed for patients with LQT2 who exhibit mutation of the KCNH2 gene. KCNH2 function is highly dependent on the extracellular potassium. It has been suggested that potassium administration will increase serum potassium level and improve repolarization abnormalities. Two small studies have shown that potassium supplements and spironolactone are associated with a significant shortening of the QTc [24, 25]. Unfortunately, there are no data that potassium supplements or spironolactone can decrease the risk of cardiac events.

Sodium Channel Blockers

Over the last decade, sodium channel blockers such as mexilitine and flecainide have been investigated as a potential treatment option for patients with LQT3. Both Mexilitine [26] and Flecainide [27–31] administration are associated with significant shortening of the QT interval among LQT3 patients.

Technical Aspects

QTc values The normal and prolonged QTc values depend on age and gender. Suggested QTc values for diagnosing QTc prolongation are: QTc >460 ms during childhood (ages 1–15 years), QTc >450 ms for adult males, and QTc >470 ms for adult females [32].

QT and QTc measurement The QT interval should be determined as a mean value derived from at least 3–5 cardiac cycles, and is measured from the beginning of the QRS complex to the end of the T wave.

The QT measurement should be made in leads II and V5 or V6, with the longest value being used. The main difficulty lies when there are T and U waves that are close together. When

T-wave deflections of a near-equal amplitude result in a biphasic T wave, the QT interval is measured to the time of final return to baseline. If a second low amplitude repolarization wave interrupts the terminal portion of the T wave, it is difficult to determine whether the second deflection is a biphasic T wave or an early-occurring U wave. In such cases, it is best to record both the QT (measured at the end of the first deflection) and the QTU (measured at the end of the second deflection) intervals [32].

The Bazett formula is widely used to correct the QT interval for heart rate (QTc); QTc equals QT divided by the square root of the R-R interval (all intervals should be measured in seconds).

Epinephrine QT stress test This provocative test may aid in unmasking individuals with concealed LQT1 [8]. There are two available protocols: by bolus infusion (Shimizu protocol) or an incremental, escalating infusion (Mayo protocol). According to the Mayo protocol [8], after 10 min of rest, 12 lead ECG recording speed was set at 50 mm/s, baseline parameters were obtained (including QT and QTc), and then an infusion of epinephrine was initiated at 0.025 µg/kg/min. After 10 min of the infusion, the measurements were repeated. The epinephrine infusion was then increased sequentially to 0.05, and 0.1 µg/kg/min, and the measurements were repeated 5 min after each dose increase. The epinephrine infusion was then discontinued, and measurements were obtained 5 and 10 min afterwards. A paradoxical response characterized by uncorrected QT lengthening (ΔQT $\geq$30 ms) rather than expected shortening appears diagnostic for LQT1 (with a sensitivity and specificity of 92 and 86 %, respectively).

Brugada Syndrome

Incidence and Etiology

Brugada syndrome is another familial disorder with structurally normal heart that involves mutations in genes encoding myocyte ion channels. Brugada syndrome is characterized by a specific ECG pattern of coved-type ST-segment elevation in the right precordial leads (V1 through V3) accompanied by a susceptibility to polymorphic VT and SCD [33]. Brugada syndrome prevalence has been estimated at 1 per 2,000 people worldwide. The prevalence is higher in Southeast Asian countries, especially Thailand, Philippines and Japan [34, 35].

Brugada syndrome is typically inherited through an autosomal dominant mode of transmission. To date, 12 Brugada syndrome-associated genes have been reported [35], with all mutations leading to either a decrease in the inward sodium or calcium current or an increase in outward potassium current.

Approximately 25 % of cases of Brugada syndrome result from mutations in the SCN5A gene that encodes for the α subunit of the cardiac sodium channel. Overall, the genetic cause has been identified for only 30 % of clinically diagnosed Brugada syndrome patients.

Diagnosis

Three ECG patterns associated with Brugada syndrome were described.

Type 1 is characterized by a J point elevation ≥2 mm (0.2 mV), a coved ST-segment elevation followed by a negativeT wave. This ECG pattern is diagnostic of Brugada syndrome. Type 2 has a J point elevation ≥2 mm, ST-segment elevation has a saddleback appearance, and then either a positive or biphasic T wave. Type 3 has either a saddleback or coved appearance with a J point elevation <2 mm, and an ST-segment elevation of <1 mm.

Type 2 and type 3 ECG are not diagnostic of the Brugada syndrome.

According to the recently published expert consensus statement [3] Brugada syndrome is definitively diagnosed when a type 1 ST-segment elevation is observed either spontaneously or after intravenous administration of a sodium channel blocking agent in at least one of the precordial leads V1 and V2, which are placed in the 2nd, 3rd or 4th intercostal space.

Brugada syndrome is diagnosed in patients with type 2 or type 3 ST-segment elevation in ≥1 lead among the precordial leads V1, V2 positioned in the 2nd, 3rd or 4th intercostal space when intravenous administration of a sodium channel blocking agent induces a type I ECG pattern.

Due to the low diagnostic yield of genetic testing among clinically diagnosed Brugada syndrome patients (genetic abnormalities are found in about 30 %), genetic testing is not recommended in the absence of a diagnostic ECG. Genetic testing may be useful for family members of a successfully genotyped proband.

Prognosis and Risk Stratification

Brugada syndrome typically manifests during adulthood, with ventricular tachyarrhythmic events occurring at an average age of 40 years and sudden death typically occurring during rest or at sleep [34]. Brugada syndrome is 8–10 times more prevalent in males than in females. At the time of diagnosis, males are more likely than females to present with previous symptoms, a spontaneous type I ECG pattern, and VF during an electrophysiology study (EPS) [36]. Although the basis for this sex-related distinction is unknown, it has been suggested that there is some sexual differences in gene expression or function and that the more prominent potassium transient outward current (Ito) in males may contribute to the male predominance of the syndrome [37].

Currently, risk stratification in Brugada syndrome relies mainly on clinical factors. The most important clinical risk factor associated with high risk of life threatening arrhythmias is the presence of syncopal episodes in patients with a spontaneous type I ECG. Other risk factors include the presence of fragmented QRS, spontaneous atrial fibrillation, and ventricular effective refractory period <200 ms during an EPS [38].

There is controversy regarding the value of programmed electrical stimulation during an EPS in predicting the risk for cardiac events. Brugada et al. [39] have found that inducibility of ventricular arrhythmias is a marker of a poor prognosis by multivariate analysis, but in both the PRELUDE (Programmed electrical stimulation predictive value) [38] and the FINGER (France, Italy, Netherlands, GERmany) [40] registries, inducibility of sustained ventricular arrhythmias did not predict ventricular arrhythmic events by multivariate analysis. Family history of SCD was not found to be an independent risk factor for cardiac events.

There are limited data on how knowledge of the Brugada syndrome specific mutation may assist in risk stratification. The presence of an SCN5A mutation has not been proven to be a risk marker in Brugada syndrome, but non-missense mutations that result in a truncated protein or missense mutations with greater than 90 % I_{Na} reduction have been found to predict syncopal episodes [41].

Management

The treatment of Brugada syndrome consists of lifestyle changes, ICD implantation and possibly medical therapy with Quinidine.

The expert consensus statement [3] recommends three lifestyle modifications for all patients with a diagnosis of Brugada syndrome: (1) avoidance of drugs that may induce or aggravate ST-segment elevation in the right precordial leads (avoiding some Ia and Ic antiarrhythmic drugs, several psychotropic drugs, and several anesthetics/ analgesics including Propofol); (2) avoidance of excessive alcohol intake; and (3) immediate treatment of fever with antipyretic drugs.

ICD implantation is recommended for patients with a history of aborted cardiac arrest or spontaneous sustained VT for secondary prevention of SCD (class I indication). ICD can be useful for patients with a spontaneous type I ECG who have a history of syncope believed to result from VT. (Class IIa indication)

ICD implantation may be considered (Class IIb indication) in patients with Brugada syndrome and inducible VF during EPS.

Quinidine can be useful in patients who qualify for an ICD but have a contraindication for ICD implantation or refuse implantation. (Class IIa)

Quinidine may be considered (Class IIb) in asymptomatic patients with Brugada syndrome who have spontaneous type I ECG.

Patients with Brugada syndrome who experience arrhythmic storms (2 or more VT/VF episodes in 24 h) may be treated by quinidine, Isopreterenol (class IIa) or by catheter ablation targeting fractionated right ventricular electrograms (class IIb).

Technical Aspects

Procaineamide provocative testing This provocative test may aid in unmasking individuals with Brugada syndrome. Baseline ECG (including high precordial leads) and vital signs should be taken at baseline, than start IV Procainamide 1 g over 30 min, measure vital signs and perform ECG every 10 min, stop infusion at 30 min and repeat ECG and vital signs at 40, 60, and 90 min. When performing provocative testing with a sodium channel blocker, the infusion should be terminated when a type-1 ECG develops, premature ventricular beats or other arrhythmias develop, or the QRS widens to ≥130 % of baseline [42].

Arrhythmogenic Right Ventricular Cardiomyopathy/Dysplasia (ARVC/D)

Incidence and Etiology

ARVC/D is a genetic heart muscle disease; its true prevalence is unknown, with estimates between 1 in 2,000 and 1 in 5,000. It is characterized pathologically by fibrofatty replacement of the right ventricular (RV) myocardium. The resulting disruption of the RV myocardial architecture in

ARVC/D can lead to RV dysfunction, ventricular tachyar-rhythmias, syncope, or SCD [34].

Several studies have suggested that mutations in various components of the cardiac desmosome have important roles in the pathogenesis of ARVC/D. Desmosomes are protein complexes specialized for cell-to-cell adhesion, supporting structural stability and maintaining normal electrical conductivity through regulation of gap junctions and calcium homeostasis. Defects in components of desmosomes may predispose to myocyte detachment and death, inflammation, repair by fibrofatty tissue, and life threatening ventricular arrhythmias [35].

Eight genes have been identified that are associated with ARVC/D: plakoglobin (JUP), desmoplakin (DSP), pla-kophilin-2 (PKP2), desmoglein-2 (DSG2), desmocollin-2 (DSC2), transforming growth factor beta-3 (TGFß3), ryano-dine receptor 2 (RYR2) and TMEM. Five of these genes (plakoglobin, desmoplakin, desmoglein-2, plakophilin-2, and, desmocollin-2) encode major components of the cardiac des-mosome. Currently known mutations in these genes identify 50 % of patients with ARVC/D with the most common type of mutations reported are in the plakophilin-2 encoded gene [34].

Diagnosis

The diagnosis of ARVC/D is based on structural, histological, ECG, arrhythmic, and familial features of the disease. Abnormalities are subdivided into major and minor categories according to the specificity of their association with ARVC/D. The diagnosis of a definite ARVC/D is fulfilled by the presence of 2 major, or 1 major plus 2 minor criteria, or 4 minor criteria from different groups. According to a proposed modification of the International Task Force Criteria [34] there are six groups of criteria: (1) Global or regional dysfunction and structural alterations assessed by echocardiography, MRI or RV angiography; (2) Tissue characterization of wall assessed by endomyocardial biopsy and histopathology; (3)

Repolarization abnormalities on the ECG including inverted T waves in right precordial leads; (4) Depolarization/conduction abnormalities including Epsilon wave (low-amplitude signals between end of QRS complex to onset of the T wave in the right precordial leads) and late potentials by signal-averaged ECG; (5) Ventricular arrhythmias including nonsustained or sustained VT of left bundle-branch block morphology and presence of >500 ventricular extrasystoles per 24 h holter monitoring; (6) Identification of a pathological mutation associated with ARVC/D or family history including a history of ARVC/D in a first-degree relative, or SCD at age <35 years.

Genotype-Phenotype Correlations and Risk Stratification

ARVC/D is inherited primarily in an autosomal dominant fashion, although there are recessive forms (e.g., Naxos disease, Carvajal syndrome) that are associated with a cutaneous phenotype. ARVC/D is a progressive heart muscle disease that with time may lead to more diffuse right ventricular (RV) involvement and left ventricular abnormalities. The severity of heart failure symptoms and the risk for ventricular arrhythmias vary considerably between patients.

There is controversy whether mutations in PKP2 (the most common implicated gene) are associated with poor prognosis and greater risk for arrhythmias [43, 44].

It was suggested that carriers of multiple mutations in ARVC/D-associated genes show a greater magnitude of myocardial involvement than carriers of a single mutation [45].

Genetic testing has an important role in the diagnosis of ARVC/D among symptomatic patients (a diagnostic yield of about 50 %) and among relatives of genotype-positive patients.

Patients at increased risk for life threatening arrhythmic events include ARVC/D with extensive disease, including left ventricular involvement, history of syncope, and affected family members with SCD.

Management

Strenuous exercise should to be avoided; medical treatment with beta-blockers, sotalol, and amiodarone are commonly used, but there are no data that drug treatment improves survival in the absence of sustained ventricular arrhythmias [46].

Thus, the mainstay of treatment is ICD implantation in selected ARVC/D patients. There is consensus that patients who had sustained VT or aborted cardiac arrest should have an ICD (Class I indication) [16].

The ACC/AHA/ESC guidelines also state that ARVC/D with extensive disease, including left ventricular involvement, one or more affected family members with SCD, or syncope are at greater risk and should receive an ICD [16].

Ablation is moderately successful for VT, but combined ICD treatment is necessary regardless of outcome. Occasional patients will undergo cardiac transplantation either because of intractable arrhythmias or severe heart failure.

References

1. Schwartz PJ, Stramba-Badiale M, Crotti L, Pedrazzini M, Besana A, Bosi G, Gabbarini F, Goulene K, Insolia R, Mannarino S, Mosca F, Nespoli L, Rimini A, Rosati E, Salice P, Spazzolini C. Prevalence of the congenital long-QT syndrome. Circulation. 2009;120:1761–7.
2. Goldenberg I, Moss AJ. Long QT syndrome. J Am Coll Cardiol. 2008;51:2291–300.
3. Priori SG, Wilde AA, Horie M, Cho Y, Behr ER, Berul C, Blom N, Brugada J, Chiang CE, Huikuri H, Kannankeril P, Krahn A, Leenhardt A, Moss A, Schwartz PJ, Shimizu W, Tomaselli G, Tracy C. HRS/EHRA/APHRS Expert Consensus Statement on the Diagnosis and Management of Patients with Inherited Primary Arrhythmia Syndromes Expert Consensus Statement on Inherited Primary Arrhythmia Syndromes: Document endorsed by HRS, EHRA, and APHRS in May 2013 and by ACCF, AHA, PACES, and AEPC in June 2013. Heart Rhythm. 2013;10(12):1932–63.

4. Schwartz PJ, Moss AJ, Vincent GM, Crampton RS. Diagnostic criteria for the long QT syndrome. An update. Circulation. 1993;88:782–4.

5. Goldenberg I, Horr S, Moss AJ, Lopes CM, Barsheshet A, McNitt S, Zareba W, Andrews ML, Robinson JL, Locati EH, Ackerman MJ, Benhorin J, Kaufman ES, Napolitano C, Platonov PG, Priori SG, Qi M, Schwartz PJ, Shimizu W, Towbin JA, Vincent GM, Wilde AA, Zhang L. Risk for life-threatening cardiac events in patients with genotype-confirmed long-QT syndrome and normal-range corrected QT intervals. J Am Coll Cardiol. 2011;57:51–9.

6. Viskin S, Postema PG, Bhuiyan ZA, Rosso R, Kalman JM, Vohra JK, Guevara-Valdivia ME, Marquez MF, Kogan E, Belhassen B, Glikson M, Strasberg B, Antzelevitch C, Wilde AA. The response of the QT interval to the brief tachycardia provoked by standing: a bedside test for diagnosing long QT syndrome. J Am Coll Cardiol. 2010;55:1955–61.

7. Horner JM, Horner MM, Ackerman MJ. The diagnostic utility of recovery phase QTc during treadmill exercise stress testing in the evaluation of long QT syndrome. Heart Rhythm. 2011;8:1698–704.

8. Vyas H, Hejlik J, Ackerman MJ. Epinephrine QT stress testing in the evaluation of congenital long-QT syndrome: diagnostic accuracy of the paradoxical QT response. Circulation. 2006;113:1385–92.

9. Viskin S, Rosso R, Rogowski O, Belhassen B, Levitas A, Wagshal A, Katz A, Fourey D, Zeltser D, Oliva A, Pollevick GD, Antzelevitch C, Rozovski U. Provocation of sudden heart rate oscillation with adenosine exposes abnormal QT responses in patients with long QT syndrome: a bedside test for diagnosing long QT syndrome. Eur Heart J. 2006;27:469–75.

10. Moss AJ, Zareba W, Benhorin J, Locati EH, Hall WJ, Robinson JL, Schwartz PJ, Towbin JA, Vincent GM, Lehmann MH. ECG T-wave patterns in genetically distinct forms of the hereditary long QT syndrome. Circulation. 1995;92:2929–34.

11. Ackerman MJ, Tester DJ, Porter CJ. Swimming, a gene-specific arrhythmogenic trigger for inherited long QT syndrome. Mayo Clin Proc. 1999;74:1088–94.

12. Moss AJ, Robinson JL, Gessman L, Gillespie R, Zareba W, Schwartz PJ, Vincent GM, Benhorin J, Heilbron EL, Towbin JA, Priori SG, Napolitano C, Zhang L, Medina A, Andrews ML,

Timothy K. Comparison of clinical and genetic variables of cardiac events associated with loud noise versus swimming among subjects with the long QT syndrome. Am J Cardiol. 1999;84:876–9.

13. Costa J, Lopes CM, Barsheshet A, Moss AJ, Migdalovich D, Ouellet G, McNitt S, Polonsky S, Robinson JL, Zareba W, Ackerman MJ, Benhorin J, Kaufman ES, Platonov PG, Shimizu W, Towbin JA, Vincent GM, Wilde AA, Goldenberg I. Combined assessment of sex- and mutation-specific information for risk stratification in type 1 long QT syndrome. Heart Rhythm. 2012; 9:892–8.

14. Migdalovich D, Moss AJ, Lopes CM, Costa J, Ouellet G, Barsheshet A, McNitt S, Polonsky S, Robinson JL, Zareba W, Ackerman MJ, Benhorin J, Kaufman ES, Platonov PG, Shimizu W, Towbin JA, Vincent GM, Wilde AA, Goldenberg I. Mutation and gender-specific risk in type 2 long QT syndrome: implications for risk stratification for life-threatening cardiac events in patients with long QT syndrome. Heart Rhythm. 2011;8: 1537–43.

15. Mullally J, Goldenberg I, Moss AJ, Lopes CM, Ackerman MJ, Zareba W, McNitt S, Robinson JL, Benhorin J, Kaufman ES, Towbin JA, Barsheshet A. Risk of life-threatening cardiac events among patients with long QT syndrome and multiple mutations. Heart Rhythm. 2013;10:378–82.

16. Zipes DP, Camm AJ, Borggrefe M, Buxton AE, Chaitman B, Fromer M, Gregoratos G, Klein G, Moss AJ, Myerburg RJ, Priori SG, Quinones MA, Roden DM, Silka MJ, Tracy C, Smith Jr SC, Jacobs AK, Adams CD, Antman EM, Anderson JL, Hunt SA, Halperin JL, Nishimura R, Ornato JP, Page RL, Riegel B, Priori SG, Blanc JJ, Budaj A, Camm AJ, Dean V, Deckers JW, Despres C, Dickstein K, Lekakis J, McGregor K, Metra M, Morais J, Osterspey A, Tamargo JL, Zamorano JL. ACC/AHA/ESC 2006 guidelines for management of patients with ventricular arrhythmias and the prevention of sudden cardiac death: a report of the American College of Cardiology/American Heart Association Task Force and the European Society of Cardiology Committee for Practice Guidelines (Writing Committee to Develop Guidelines for Management of Patients With Ventricular Arrhythmias and the Prevention of Sudden Cardiac Death). J Am Coll Cardiol. 2006;48:e247–346.

17. Kim JA, Lopes CM, Moss AJ, McNitt S, Barsheshet A, Robinson JL, Zareba W, Ackerman MJ, Kaufman ES, Towbin JA, Vincent

M, Goldenberg I. Trigger-specific risk factors and response to therapy in long QT syndrome type 2. Heart Rhythm. 2010;7:1797–805.

18. Schwartz PJ, Priori SG, Spazzolini C, Moss AJ, Vincent GM, Napolitano C, Denjoy I, Guicheney P, Breithardt G, Keating MT, Towbin JA, Beggs AH, Brink P, Wilde AA, Toivonen L, Zareba W, Robinson JL, Timothy KW, Corfield V, Wattanasirichaigoon D, Corbett C, Haverkamp W, Schulze-Bahr E, Lehmann MH, Schwartz K, Coumel P, Bloise R. Genotype-phenotype correlation in the long-QT syndrome: gene-specific triggers for life-threatening arrhythmias. Circulation. 2001;103:89–95.

19. Moss AJ, Zareba W, Hall WJ, Schwartz PJ, Crampton RS, Benhorin J, Vincent GM, Locati EH, Priori SG, Napolitano C, Medina A, Zhang L, Robinson JL, Timothy K, Towbin JA, Andrews ML. Effectiveness and limitations of beta-blocker therapy in congenital long-QT syndrome. Circulation. 2000;101:616–23.

20. Goldenberg I, Bradley J, Moss A, McNitt S, Polonsky S, Robinson JL, Andrews M, Zareba W. Beta-blocker efficacy in high-risk patients with the congenital long-QT syndrome types 1 and 2: implications for patient management. J Cardiovasc Electrophysiol. 2010;21:893–901.

21. Barsheshet A, Goldenberg I, O-Uchi J, Moss AJ, Jons C, Shimizu W, Wilde AA, McNitt S, Peterson DR, Zareba W, Robinson JL, Ackerman MJ, Cypress M, Gray DA, Hofman N, Kanters JK, Kaufman ES, Platonov PG, Qi M, Towbin JA, Vincent GM, Lopes CM. Mutations in cytoplasmic loops of the KCNQ1 channel and the risk of life-threatening events: implications for mutation-specific response to beta-blocker therapy in type 1 long-QT syndrome. Circulation. 2012;125:1988–96.

22. Matavel A, Medei E, Lopes CM. PKA and PKC partially rescue long QT type 1 phenotype by restoring channel-PIP(2) interactions. Channels (Austin). 2010;4.

23. Chockalingam P, Crotti L, Girardengo G, Johnson JN, Harris KM, van der Heijden JF, Hauer RN, Beckmann BM, Spazzolini C, Rordorf R, Rydberg A, Clur SA, Fischer M, van den Heuvel F, Kaab S, Blom NA, Ackerman MJ, Schwartz PJ, Wilde AA. Not all beta-blockers are equal in the management of long QT syndrome types 1 and 2: higher recurrence of events under metoprolol. J Am Coll Cardiol. 2012;60:2092–9.

24. Compton SJ, Lux RL, Ramsey MR, Strelich KR, Sanguinetti MC, Green LS, Keating MT, Mason JW. Genetically defined

therapy of inherited long-QT syndrome. Correction of abnormal repolarization by potassium. Circulation. 1996;94:1018–22.

25. Etheridge SP, Compton SJ, Tristani-Firouzi M, Mason JW. A new oral therapy for long QT syndrome: long-term oral potassium improves repolarization in patients with HERG mutations. J Am Coll Cardiol. 2003;42:1777–82.

26. Schwartz PJ, Priori SG, Locati EH, Napolitano C, Cantu F, Towbin JA, Keating MT, Hammoude H, Brown AM, Chen LS. Long QT syndrome patients with mutations of the SCN5A and HERG genes have differential responses to Na+ channel blockade and to increases in heart rate. Implications for gene-specific therapy. Circulation. 1995;92:3381–6.

27. Nagatomo T, January CT, Makielski JC. Preferential block of late sodium current in the LQT3 DeltaKPQ mutant by the class I(C) antiarrhythmic flecainide. Mol Pharmacol. 2000;57:101–7.

28. Windle JR, Geletka RC, Moss AJ, Zareba W, Atkins DL. Normalization of ventricular repolarization with flecainide in long QT syndrome patients with SCN5A:DeltaKPQ mutation. Ann Noninvasive Electrocardiol. 2001;6:153–8.

29. Moss AJ, Windle JR, Hall WJ, Zareba W, Robinson JL, McNitt S, Severski P, Rosero S, Daubert JP, Qi M, Cieciorka M, Manalan AS. Safety and efficacy of flecainide in subjects with Long QT-3 syndrome (DeltaKPQ mutation): a randomized, double-blind, placebo-controlled clinical trial. Ann Noninvasive Electrocardiol. 2005;10:59–66.

30. Stokoe KS, Balasubramaniam R, Goddard CA, Colledge WH, Grace AA, Huang CL. Effects of flecainide and quinidine on arrhythmogenic properties of Scn5a+/− murine hearts modelling the Brugada syndrome. J Physiol. 2007;581:255–75.

31. Anno T, Hondeghem LM. Interactions of flecainide with guinea pig cardiac sodium channels. Importance of activation unblocking to the voltage dependence of recovery. Circ Res. 1990;66:789–803.

32. Goldenberg I, Moss AJ, Zareba W. QT interval: how to measure it and what is "normal". J Cardiovasc Electrophysiol. 2006;17:333–6.

33. Brugada P, Brugada J. Right bundle branch block, persistent ST segment elevation and sudden cardiac death: a distinct clinical and electrocardiographic syndrome. A multicenter report. J Am Coll Cardiol. 1992;20:1391–6.

34. Marcus FI, McKenna WJ, Sherrill D, Basso C, Bauce B, Bluemke DA, Calkins H, Corrado D, Cox MG, Daubert JP, Fontaine G,

Gear K, Hauer R, Nava A, Picard MH, Protonotarios N, Saffitz JE, Sanborn DM, Steinberg JS, Tandri H, Thiene G, Towbin JA, Tsatsopoulou A, Wichter T, Zareba W. Diagnosis of arrhythmogenic right ventricular cardiomyopathy/dysplasia: proposed modification of the task force criteria. Circulation. 2010; 121:1533–41.

35. Awad MM, Calkins H, Judge DP. Mechanisms of disease: molecular genetics of arrhythmogenic right ventricular dysplasia/cardiomyopathy. Nat Clin Pract Cardiovasc Med. 2008;5:258–67.

36. Benito B, Sarkozy A, Mont L, Henkens S, Berruezo A, Tamborero D, Arzamendi D, Berne P, Brugada R, Brugada P, Brugada J. Gender differences in clinical manifestations of Brugada syndrome. J Am Coll Cardiol. 2008;52:1567–73.

37. Marcus FI, Zareba W, Calkins H, Towbin JA, Basso C, Bluemke DA, Estes 3rd NA, Picard MH, Sanborn D, Thiene G, Wichter T, Cannom D, Wilber DJ, Scheinman M, Duff H, Daubert J, Talajic M, Krahn A, Sweeney M, Garan H, Sakaguchi S, Lerman BB, Kerr C, Kron J, Steinberg JS, Sherrill D, Gear K, Brown M, Severski P, Polonsky S, McNitt S. Arrhythmogenic right ventricular cardiomyopathy/dysplasia clinical presentation and diagnostic evaluation: results from the North American Multidisciplinary Study. Heart Rhythm. 2009;6:984–92.

38. Priori SG, Gasparini M, Napolitano C, Della Bella P, Ottonelli AG, Sassone B, Giordano U, Pappone C, Mascioli G, Rossetti G, De Nardis R, Colombo M. Risk stratification in Brugada syndrome: results of the PRELUDE (PRogrammed ELectrical stimUlation preDictive valuE) registry. J Am Coll Cardiol. 2012;59:37–45.

39. Brugada J, Brugada R, Brugada P. Determinants of sudden cardiac death in individuals with the electrocardiographic pattern of Brugada syndrome and no previous cardiac arrest. Circulation. 2003;108:3092–6.

40. Probst V, Veltmann C, Eckardt L, Meregalli PG, Gaita F, Tan HL, Babuty D, Sacher F, Giustetto C, Schulze-Bahr E, Borggrefe M, Haissaguerre M, Mabo P, Le Marec H, Wolpert C, Wilde AA. Long-term prognosis of patients diagnosed with Brugada syndrome: results from the FINGER Brugada Syndrome Registry. Circulation. 2010;121:635–43.

41. Meregalli PG, Tan HL, Probst V, Koopmann TT, Tanck MW, Bhuiyan ZA, Sacher F, Kyndt F, Schott JJ, Albuisson J, Mabo P, Bezzina CR, Le Marec H, Wilde AA. Type of SCN5A mutation determines clinical severity and degree of conduction slowing in

190 A. Barsheshet and I. Goldenberg

loss-of-function sodium channelopathies. Heart Rhythm. 2009;6:341–8.

42. Obeyesekere MN, Klein GJ, Modi S, Leong-Sit P, Gula LJ, Yee R, Skanes AC, Krahn AD. How to perform and interpret provocative testing for the diagnosis of Brugada syndrome, long-QT syndrome, and catecholaminergic polymorphic ventricular tachycardia. Circ Arrhythm Electrophysiol. 2011;4:958–64.

43. Dalal D, Molin LH, Piccini J, Tichnell C, James C, Bomma C, Prakasa K, Towbin JA, Marcus FI, Spevak PJ, Bluemke DA, Abraham T, Russell SD, Calkins H, Judge DP. Clinical features of arrhythmogenic right ventricular dysplasia/cardiomyopathy associated with mutations in plakophilin-2. Circulation. 2006;113:1641–9.

44. van Tintelen JP, Entius MM, Bhuiyan ZA, Jongbloed R, Wiesfeld AC, Wilde AA, van der Smagt J, Boven LG, Mannens MM, van Langen IM, Hofstra RM, Otterspoor LC, Doevendans PA, Rodriguez LM, van Gelder IC, Hauer RN. Plakophilin-2 mutations are the major determinant of familial arrhythmogenic right ventricular dysplasia/cardiomyopathy. Circulation. 2006;113:1650–8.

45. Bauce B, Nava A, Beffagna G, Basso C, Lorenzon A, Smaniotto G, De Bortoli M, Rigato I, Mazzotti E, Steriotis A, Marra MP, Towbin JA, Thiene G, Danieli GA, Rampazzo A. Multiple mutations in desmosomal proteins encoding genes in arrhythmogenic right ventricular cardiomyopathy/dysplasia. Heart Rhythm. 2010;7:22–9.

46. Smith W. Guidelines for the diagnosis and management of arrhythmogenic right ventricular cardiomyopathy. Heart Lung Circ. 2011;20:757–60.

47. Barsheshet A, Dotsenko O, Goldenberg I. Genotype-specific risk stratification and management of patients with long QT syndrome. Ann Noninvasive Electrocardiol. 2013;18(6):499–509.

Index

D.T. Huang, T. Prinzi (eds.), *Clinical Cardiac Electrophysiology in Clinical Practice*, In Clinical Practice, DOI 10.1007/978-1-4471-5433-4, © Springer-Verlag London 2015

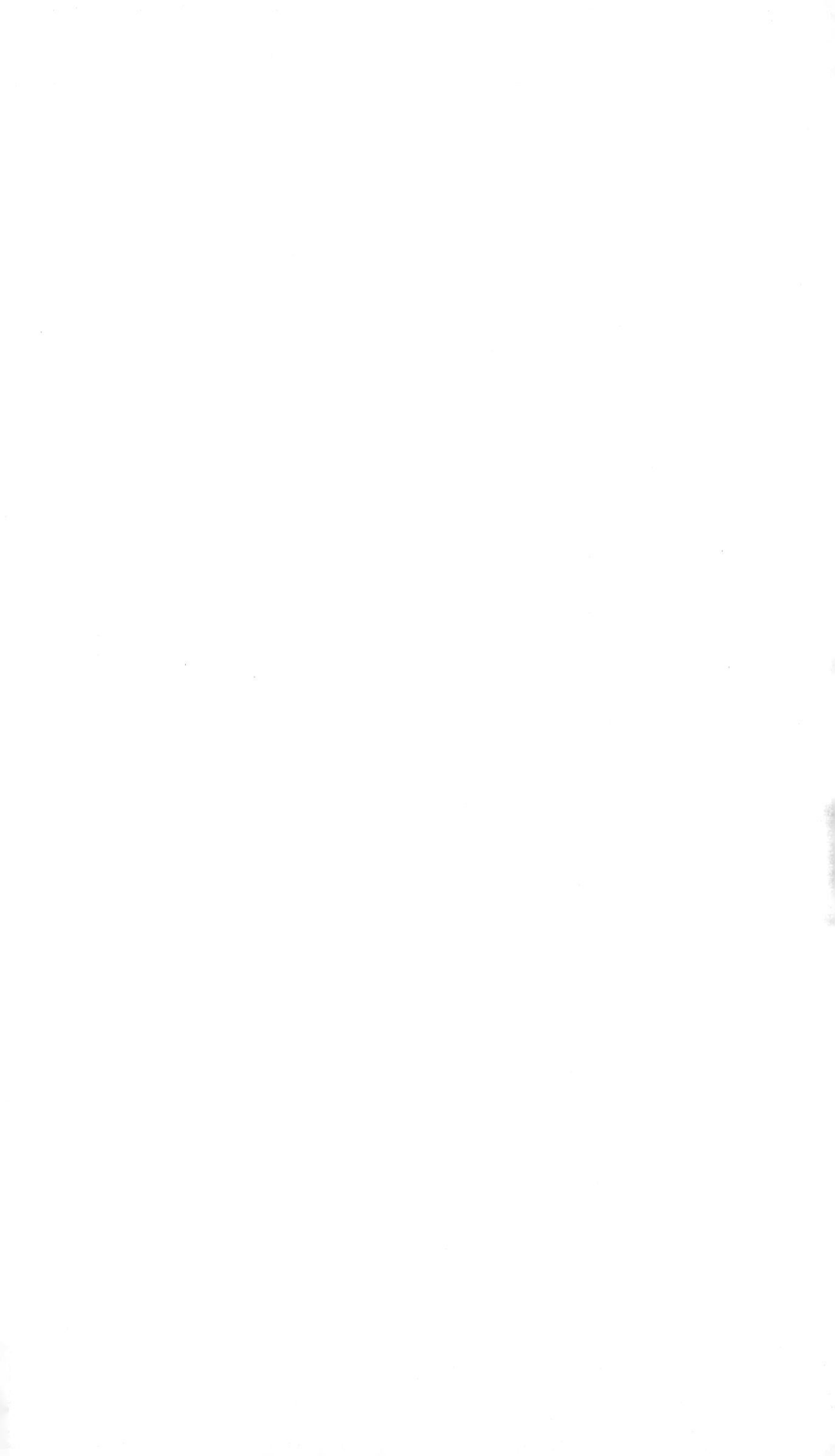

Printed by Printforce, the Netherlands

In Clinical Practice

David T. Huang · Travis Prinzi *Editors*

Clinical Cardiac Electrophysiology in Clinical Practice

This is a practical guide to the clinical diagnosis and treatment of cardiac arrhythmias that meets the needs of this highly specialized, complex and growing field of cardiology. As understanding of the evaluation of treatment of arrhythmias continues to advance, learning and understanding the principles of electrophysiology in order to provide the best possible treatments for patients can be a daunting task.

With a scientific, practical, and multi-disciplinary approach, *Clinical Cardiac Electrophysiology in Clinical Practice* establishes the foundation of the subject and provides a concise illustrative approach to facilitate and enhance understanding. It is designed to be accessible to serve as an introduction to electrophysiology, but advanced enough to serve as a guide for experienced practitioners. Electrophysiology students of all levels, including residents, fellows, mid-level providers, nurses, technologists, primary care providers, cardiologists and electrophysiologists will find value in these pages.

Cardiology

ISBN 978-1-4471-5432-7

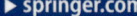

▶ springer.com